Current Clinical Practice

D1563665

Series Editor
Neil S. Skolnik
Temple University, School of Medicine, Abington Memorial Hospital,
Jenkintown, PA, USA

For further volumes:
http://www.springer.com/series/7633

Neil S. Skolnik • Amy Lynn Clouse
Jo Ann Woodward
Editors

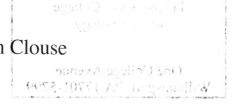

Sexually Transmitted Diseases

A Practical Guide for Primary Care

Second Edition

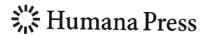 Humana Press

Editors
Neil S. Skolnik, MD
Abington Family Medicine
Abington Memorial Hospital
Jenkintown, PA, USA

Amy Lynn Clouse, MD
Abington Family Medicine
Abington Memorial Hospital
Jenkintown, PA, USA

Jo Ann Woodward, MHI, WHNP-BC
Scottsdale, AZ, USA

ISBN 978-1-62703-498-2   ISBN 978-1-62703-499-9 (eBook)
DOI 10.1007/978-1-62703-499-9
Springer New York Heidelberg Dordrecht London

Library of Congress Control Number: 2013939596

Printed on acid-free paper

Humana Press is a brand of Springer
Springer is part of Springer Science+Business Media (www.springer.com)

Preface

A valuable approach to providing excellent care of patients with sexually transmitted diseases requires that primary care physicians integrate detailed knowledge and clinical wisdom along with empathy to provide care of patients for one of the most emotionally difficult diseases any person encounters during his or her lifetime. STDs are common; they account for 5 % of all outpatient office visits in the United States, and are primarily managed by family doctors, internists, obstetrician-gynecologists, emergency room physicians, primary care nurse practitioners, and physician assistants. Four of the top five reportable infectious diseases in the United States are STDs [1]. In fact, one in ten Americans will have an STD at some time during his or her life [2]. STDs are unique in that they are defined not by their symptoms, or by the body organs that they infect, or by the microorganisms that cause infection, but rather by their mode of transmission—primarily through sexual intercourse. While STDs are related through their mode of transmission, they are heterogeneous and their effects on the body, causing illness that ranges from limited, localized, and asymptomatic disease to serious systemic acute and chronic illness.

STDs reflect the intersection of public health with private decision making and the actions and consequences that ensue from those decisions. Because of their mode of transmission, and the fact that what is inherently a private activity has direct public health consequences, prevention, screening, and treatment of STDs must occur as a part of public discourse as well as private discussions between clinicians and their patients. Unlike most other diseases and infections, the diagnosis of an STD often carries with it a stigma of guilt and embarrassment. This can make the discussion about the mode of acquisition and future prevention difficult for patients and practitioners, resulting in less than optimal communication, misinformation, increased psychosocial burden and the risk of increased disease transmission into the future.

Discussing sexual behavior can be an embarrassing experience that is often avoided by the patient and the practitioner. We as practitioners carry certain biases, recognized or not. These are obvious obstacles to excellent care. The practitioner's approach, however, can change the experience of a patient from embarrassing or even shameful into an opportunity to empower themselves with knowledge and behavioral change that may save their life. STDs should be handled candidly and honestly, with empathy for the psychosocial ramifications of the illness and an eye toward the possibility of personal growth and modifications of behavior.

The history of STDs is informative. STDs were long ago recognized as being spread by sexual contact, and where therefore referred to as "*venereal diseases*," named after the Greek goddess of love, Venus. Individuals who had syphilis were shunned. Until the 1960s, syphilis and gonorrhea were the only STDs. During the 1970s Chlamydia trachomatis became recognized as causing urethritis, cervicitis, and pelvic inflammatory disease (PID). During the 1980s, HSV-2 appeared to be almost epidemic, and was in fact thought, incorrectly, to be the etiologic agent for cervical cancer. Also during the 1980s the acquired immunodeficiency virus (AIDS) was identified with the human immunodeficiency virus (HIV) being identified as the etiologic agent. During the early part of the AIDS epidemic, paralleling the history of the syphilis epidemic, biases against groups felt to transmit the virus were common [3]. In the latter part of the 1980s and 1990s the role of the sexually transmitted Human Papilloma Virus (HPV) in the development of cervical cancer was recognized, culminating in the development of HPV vaccine, the first vaccine thought to prevent the development of cancer [2].

STDs in the United States continue to be an important public health challenge. There were over 1.3 million cases of chlamydia infections reported in 2010, for a rate of 426.0 per 100,000 population, which represents the highest rate of any infection reportable to the CDC and was a 5.1 % increase compared to the previous year. Chlamydia infections are usually asymptomatic in women but can lead to PID and subsequent infertility, ectopic pregnancy, and chronic pelvic pain. Rates in women were more than twice that of men in 2010, partially due to the increased rates of screening. Racial and ethnic disparities were clear; the chlamydia rate in blacks was 8 times that in whites [1].

In contrast to chlamydia, gonorrhea infection reached its lowest rate ever in 2009. Rates dropped to 98.1 per 100,000 from a high of over 464 per 100,000 population in 1975. 2010 saw a slight increase to 100.8 per 100,000 population. Gonorrhea is a significant cause of PID but, despite the overall decline in infection rates, treatment is becoming more difficult. The *Gonococcal Isolate Surveillance Project* from the CDC in 2012 showed increasing gonococcal resistance to cephalosporins, to the point where oral cephalosporins are no longer recommended as treatment [4].

The rate of reported primary and secondary syphilis in the United States was at an historic low of approximately 11 per 100,000 between 2000 and 2005. A concerning trend, however, has developed recently with the rate climbing by over one-third to 14.9 per 100,00 in 2010, most marked in men who have sex with men.

As mentioned above, new technology is emerging with the most important example being the human papillomavirus vaccine and the probability of decreased development of cervical cancer. The CDC's Advisory Committee on Immunization Practices (ACIP) in 2006 recommended vaccination of girls starting at age 11–12, and in 2011 recommended routine vaccination of males age 11–12.

Addressing STDs adequately requires individual practitioners with a detailed understanding of STDs to see patients with both knowledge and empathy as a primary directive, as well as a public health approach for disease surveillance, detection, and treatment. Working to eliminate the stigma of STDs by engaging in frank discussions about symptoms and sexual behavior, screening for appropriate STDs in the appropriate setting, and continuing to profess the message of responsible sexual decision making puts primary care physicians in a unique position to carry out prevention, detection, and treatment of sexually transmitted diseases.

Jenkintown, PA, USA   Neil S. Skolnik
Jenkintown, PA, USA   Amy Lynn Clouse
Abington, PA, USA   Curtis Olson

References

1. Centers for Disease Control and Prevention. [Summary of Notifiable Diseases, 2010]. Published 1 June 2012 for MMWR. 2010;59(No. 53):[inclusive page numbers].
2. Nelson A. Introduction to sexually transmitted infections—a view of the past and an assessment of present challenges in current clinical practice: sexually transmitted diseases. A practical guide for primary care. Totowa, NJ: Humana Press; 2008.
3. Shilts R. And the band played on: politics, people, and the AIDS epidemic, 20th-Anniversary edition. St. Martin's Griffin; Revised edition; 2007.
4. CDC. Update to CDC's sexually transmitted diseases treatment guidelines, 2010: oral cephalosporins no longer a recommended treatment for gonococcal infections. MMWR. 2012;61(31):590–94.

Acknowledgements

A book can be like a wild flower caught out of the corner of one's eye while walking down a winding path. What begins as a surprise takes form as one looks more closely. Then as astonishment shifts to appreciation it can take one on an unanticipated journey. In that way, a book is like life, never certain, but filled with unanticipated challenges that have to be reckoned with through patience and cooperation with others. This book on sexually transmitted diseases came upon us as such a surprise and we have learned many things in the course of its writing. One of the things that we, the editors, learned again was how fortunate we are to work in an environment where learners of all levels—medical students, residents, and attending physicians—work together to provide excellent care for patients, and how we are able to combine the joys and challenges of patient care with the intellectual excitement of putting information together, in this case in the form of a book.

In writing this book, Amy and Neil are reminded of our good fortune to be working with smart, fun, inquisitive, supportive colleagues—Mat Clark, Adam Chrusch, Trip Hansen, Natalie McGann, John Russell, and Meera Shah. We have together, along with the support of many team players including Joyce Westaby and Muriel Wimpenny, been able to develop a family medicine residency program that integrates the best aspects of clinical and academic medicine in an outstanding and enjoyable manner. A residency program like this, that sees patients from all backgrounds regardless of their ability to pay in an environment of support and respect, can only occur when supported strongly by a parent hospital and the people who are in charge of that hospital—Larry Merlis, Jack Kelly, Meg McGoldrick, and many others—all of whom share a commitment to doing the right thing—providing high quality, safe, compassionate medical care to the patients in our community.

The joys of life, whether it is writing a book or spotting a wild flower during a walk, have much less meaning when they are not shared. We feel lucky to be able to share our appreciation and thanks with both our professional and our personal families. Our professional families are mentioned above. Our personal families follow. Neil's appreciation goes to Alison, Aaron, and Ava each of whom know they hold a special wild place in his heart. Amy's appreciation goes to her family and friends who continue to remind her to live with grace and take herself a little less seriously,

seriously. Jo Ann's appreciation is given to Linda Caryn Goldman and the multidis-ciplinary team approach that this book reflects. Representing different disciplines of healthcare providers is part of the integrative nature of this book.

We hope that you find this book useful and informative.

Jenkintown, PA, USA   Neil S. Skolnik
Jenkintown, PA, USA   Amy Lynn Clouse
Scottsdale, AZ, USA   Jo Ann Woodward

Contents

Contributors

Joshua H. Barash Department of Family and Community Medicine, Thomas Jefferson University Hospital, Philadelphia, PA, USA

Edward Buchanan Department of Family and Community Medicine, Thomas Jefferson University, Philadelphia, PA, USA

Mathew M. Clark Family Medicine Residency Program, Abington Memorial Hospital, Jenkintown, PA, USA

Amy Lynn Clouse Abington Family Medicine, Abington Memorial Hospital, Jenkintown, PA, USA

Linda Caryn Goldman School of Nursing, California State University Dominguez Hills, Carson, CA, USA

Jeremy Herman Department of Medicine, Division of Gastroenterology, Cedars Sinai Medical Center, Beverly Hills, CA, USA

Christina Hillson Department of Family and Community Medicine, Thomas Jefferson University, Philadelphia, PA, USA

Elissa Meites Division of STD Prevention, Centers for Disease Control and Prevention, Atlanta, GA, USA

Anne Moore School of Nursing, Vanderbilt University, Nashville, TN, USA

D. Gene Parks Department of Obstetrics and Gynecology, David Geffen School of Medicine at UCLA, Los Angeles, CA, USA

Albert John Phillips Obstetrics & Gynecology, Keck School of Medicine, University of Southern California, Los Angeles, CA, USA

Justin A. Reynolds Division of Digestive Diseases, Department of Medicine, David Geffen School of Medicine at UCLA, Los Angeles, CA, USA

Gunter Rieg Kaiser Permanente Medical Group, Medicine Department, David Geffen School of Medicine at UCLA, Harbor City, CA, USA

Department of Medicine, Division of Infectious Diseases, Kaiser Permanente South Bay Medical Center, Harbor City, CA, USA

Neil S. Skolnik Abington Family Medicine, Abington Memorial Hospital, Jenkintown, PA, USA

Christine M. Stroka Family Medicine Residency Program, Abington Memorial Hospital, Jenkintown, PA, USA

Mafudia Suaray Department of Family and Community Medicine, Thomas Jefferson University, Philadelphia, PA, USA

Carolyn M. Sutton Department of Obstetrics and Gynecology, University of Texas Southwestern Medical Center at Dallas, Dallas, TX, USA

Jennifer E. Thuener Family Medicine, Abington Memorial Hospital, Jenkintown, PA, USA

Jo Ann Woodward Scottsdale, AZ, USA

Kimberly A. Workowski Division of STD Prevention, Centers for Disease Control and Prevention, Atlanta, GA, USA

Department of Medicine, Infectious Diseases, Emory University, Atlanta, GA, USA

Chapter 1
Human Papillomavirus and Genital Warts

Linda Caryn Goldman and Amy Lynn Clouse

Introduction

Unknown until the second half of the twentieth century, human papillomavirus (HPV) is now recognized as being one of the most common sexually transmitted infections (STI) in the United States, accounting for more than one third of the new cases of STIs each year [1]. Most HPV infections cause no symptoms, other types can cause genital warts, and still others cause invasive squamous cell anogenital carcinoma. This chapter provides an overview of HPV infection—its transmissibility and epidemiology. It focuses on genital warts in its discussion of the clinical consequences of HPV infection and treatment options. The contribution HPV infection makes to various genital cancers is mentioned, but the screening, diagnosis, and treatments of these conditions are outside the scope of this book.

Prevalence/Incidence

Precise estimates of the incidence of HPV infection are not available for several reasons. First, HPV is not a reportable disease. Additionally, most infections are subclinical. Of the patients who develop findings with HPV infection, most have

L.C. Goldman, MSN, WHNP-BC, FNP (✉)
School of Nursing, California State University Dominguez Hills,
1000 E. Victoria St., Carson, CA 90747, USA
e-mail: lindagfnp@yahoo.com; lgoldman@csudh.edu

A.L. Clouse, MD
Abington Family Medicine, Abington Memorial Hospital, Jenkintown,
PA 19046, USA

N.S. Skolnik et al. (eds.), *Sexually Transmitted Diseases: A Practical Guide for Primary Care*, Current Clinical Practice, DOI 10.1007/978-1-62703-499-9_1,
© Springer Science+Business Media New York 2013

only indirect indication of infections, such as abnormal cervical cytology. In patients who have more obvious manifestations of infection, such as external genital warts, no formal testing is done to document the presence of HPV. Finally, HPV also causes recurrent outbreaks of lesions. Because most first infections are asymptomatic, it may be difficult to recognize new cases from recurrent infections, which must be done to calculate incidence.

Prevalence of HPV infection is also difficult to estimate. The usual technique used to estimate the number of people infected with HPV is to measure serum antibodies. However, most people who acquire the viral infection clear that infection within 1–2 years; others may harbor the infection for years without outbreaks; others will have obvious recurrences. Some people in these groups will have positive antibody titers, so that antibodies may overstate the number of people who are currently infected (prevalence) [2]. Confusing the situation even further is the fact that only 50 % of individuals infected with HPV will develop detectable antibody titers to the virus, which could underestimate prevalence.

Despite these limitations, several studies performed over the past 20 years have demonstrated a steady rise in the number of new cases of genital HPV. The number of office visits for genital HPV disease has increased over the last 30 years [3]. It has been estimated that about 15 % (20–24 million) of adults in the United States are currently infected with this virus; 9.2 million of them are between the ages of 15 and 24 years [4–6]. The prevalence of HPV infection among sexually active college women over a 3-year period has been reported to be over 40 %; the greatest prevalence is among women with 3 or more lifetime partners or partners with 2 or more lifetime sexual partners [7–9].

Risk Factors

Acquisition of HPV is clearly related to sexual activity. The highest risk groups for new infection are sexually active adolescents under the age of 19, followed by adults aged 19–30 [10]. The risk of HPV infection increases with number of lifetime sex partners. In one study, patients with 10 or more partners were found to have 58 % current infection rates compared with an 8 % rate in those with zero or one partner [11]. Risk factors for HPV acquisition are similar to those for other STIs, and include multiple recent sex partners and changing sex partners in the last year. Coinfection with other STDs and early age at first intercourse increase the risk of HPV infection. Expression of the virus and clearance of viral infection are related to immunocompetence of the host. Human immunodeficiency virus (HIV) infection increases the risk of HPV infection and the risk of developing HPV-related disease. All of the factors that predispose to persistent infection (those infections that do not clear) have not been elucidated. Persistent infections are associated with recurrent wart outbreaks and increase the risk of HPV-related malignancy.

Infectivity and Transmission

HPV is most commonly transmitted during sexual activity, which involves skin-to-skin contact; microabrasions in the area of contact permit the virus to be transmitted from one sexual partner to another. Even in the absence of visible lesions, such as a genital wart, the microabrasions expose the HPV-infected cells in the basal epithelium of the host and increase viral shedding. More importantly, microabrasions in the recipient expose vulnerable basal epithelial cells to the virus. About 60–66 % of sex partners of HPV-infected people will develop detectable HPV lesions, although they may be very subtle appearing or may be located in areas that escape normal detection [12]. About 50–55 % of men whose partners have cervical HPV disease have HPV-associated penile lesions [13]. HPV can also be transmitted from one woman to another [14].

Oral–genital contact can transmit infection. Early studies suggested that about 4 % of women with external genital warts also had buccal lesions. High-risk HPV has been found in about 25 % of oral cancers, supporting hypothesis there is some transmission via that route [15].

Perianal infection is quite common. Transmission is possible in men and women who have anal receptive sex with men. However, the presence of genital warts around the anus does not necessarily indicate a history of receptive anal intercourse. In one study, only 10 % of women who shed HPV from the anal area admitted to having anal intercourse, and 83 % of those with virus in the anal area, were also positive for HPV in cervical, vulvar, and vaginal samples [16].

The virus can also be transmitted by fomites. Transmission of the virus to the anogenital area has been reported in tanning beds and saunas. Other nondirect transmission may be possible via sex toys, exam tables, door knobs, and contamination of exam lights adjusted by examining hands [17].

Vertical transmission from mother to her newborn is possible, though rare, during delivery through an HPV-infected birth canal. The most serious complication that occurs for the newborn is respiratory/laryngeal papillomatosis. Genital warts and facial lesions in the infant can also result from exposure during delivery. However, it is not yet clear that cesarean delivery prevents HPV transmission to the baby and should only be performed if genital warts obstruct the birth canal.

Etiology

Papillomaviruses infect many animal species including cotton-tail rabbits, cattle, and humans. They are named and classified by their natural host. More than 120 different types of *human* papillomaviruses have been identified, but some have only been partially sequenced. HPV types are assigned new numbers when there is more than a 10 % difference in gene sequences in particular regions of the viral DNA and they

Table 1.1 Low risk vs. high risk HPV types

Low risk HPV types	High risk HPV types
Possess little to no oncogenic potential	Possess oncogenic potential
HPV 6,11,40,42,43,44,54,61,70,72,81 and CP6108	HPV 16,18,31,33,35,39,45,51,52,56,58,59, 68,73,82 and probably 26,53,66
Most commonly found on the external genitalia	Most commonly found as flat warts
Primarily responsible for external genital warts	Primarily responsible for intraepithelial neoplasias of the cervix, anus
Also responsible for juvenile respiratory papillomatosis	Also responsible for penile and anal carcinoma

Adapted from Munoz N, Bosch FX, de Sanjose S, et al. Epidemiologic classification of human papilloma-virus types associated with cervical cancer. N Engl J Med. 2003;348:518–27

are numbered in their order of discovery. All known HPV share a similar structure and genomic organization of small, non-enveloped virions with a double-stranded, circular DNA of 7800–7900 base pairs encased in an icosahedral protein capsid.

In general, genital HPV types have been classified into two groups based on the oncogenic potential—low- and intermediate/high-risk groups (*see* Table 1.1). The low-risk types (mainly 6 and 11) are responsible for almost half of the external genital warts. However, mixed viral types may be involved in the wart formation. The low-risk viral types have also been isolated from the lesions involved in laryngeal papillomatosis/respiratory papillomatosis in the tracheobronchial trees of children [18, 19]. The high-risk HPV types are primarily involved in the development of squamous cell cancerous lesions of the uterine cervix, anus, vulva, and penis [12, 20, 21], but also contribute to external genital warts. Four HPV types (6, 11, 16, and 18) account for 90 % of genital HPV infection.

Clinical Course

The usual reservoirs of genital HPV infection are the moist mucosa and adjacent squamous epithelia of the male and female genitalia, the cervix, and the anus. Microabrasions that develop during sexual activity enable the infected partner to shed virus and the uninfected partner to become more susceptible to infection. Repeated trauma in the area increases infectivity as wound healing stimulates cell division, increasing episomal viral replication [22]. The virus enters the basal epithelial cells in areas such as the inner labia minora in woman and the prepuce and frenulum in men. Anal epithelium is also traumatized easily during sex, permitting HPV infection. The virus also preferentially infects the rapidly dividing cells within the transitional zone of the cervix.

After introduction of the virus into the host basal epithelial cells, the virus sheds its protein capsule and coexists within the host cell as a circular episome. The virus then enters into a latent incubation period of 1–8 months, during which time there are no visible manifestations of the infection. The active growth phase starts when the first lesion develops. It is not known what induces the transition from latent to infective stage, but many host, viral, and environmental factors are involved. During the active infection phase, the HPV replicates independent of host cell division and induces the host cells to proliferate, creating a myriad of lesions from flat to papillary warts. Viral counts are highest in the superficial layers of the epithelium, increasing infectivity. During this phase, patients generally seek therapy.

Approximately 3 months later, the host immune system mounts a response. The innate immune system is recruited and interferons slow HPV replication and trigger the cell-mediated immune response. An immunocompetent cell-mediated immune system and cytokine production are needed for HPV clearance, but there are still challenges to viral clearance in immunocompetent hosts. HPV has some protection from the host response because the virus is intracellularly located. In addition, the epithelial cells in the perineum do not present antigens well to the host, so the HPV may not be recognized by the immune system [23]. HPV blocks the host response by depleting local intraepithelial lymphocytes, Langerhan's cells, and CD4+ cells and down regulating cytokine production [22]. However, lysis of the infected cells exposes the HPV to the host and triggers more intense defense.

About 80–90 % of people will clear the infection so that the virus can no longer be detected. Only 10–20 % of individuals will have persistent infection that can express itself either as a latent infection, which may be periodically reactivated, or as a persistent (and more difficult-to-treat) infection. Recurrences are more likely when host immune system is compromised by chemotherapy, corticosteroid therapy, or HIV infection.

Clinical Manifestations

Genital warts can be found on the external genitalia, the vagina, cervix, anus, mouth, and larynx. Most patients with genital warts are asymptomatic. In a study of university women, neither acute nor persistent HPV infection (documented by viral shedding) was associated with discharge, itching, burning, soreness, or fissure [16]. Even women with genital warts had none of the associated symptoms. Patients with external genital warts may complain of a bump or mass they palpate or see on inspection. Infected or large lesions may be tender or associated with spotting, odor, or tenderness. Larger internal warts may produce dyspareunia or postcoital spotting. Urethral lesions may impair flow of urine or ejaculate. Condyloma acuminata are the classical external genital warts. They are raised, acuminate, exophytic lesions, which on keratinized skin are white, gray, or flesh-colored warty lesions. On mucosal surfaces, low-risk HPV tends to have finger-like projections and blend in color with surrounding tissue.

Another presentation of HPV in the genital area are papillomas. Papillomas are raised, possibly pigmented lesions, which are slow-growing and sometimes pedunculated. They are often mistaken for skin tags or moles and are most commonly found on keratinized skin.

The high-risk HPV usually causes flat genital warts. They may be hyperpigmented, white or red, depending on the impact HPV has on local melanocytes.

In women, external warts may present anywhere on the vulva, perineum, and perianal area. External genital warts in men may involve the squamous epidermis of the penis, foreskin, scrotum, perineum, and perianal area. Internal warts affect the mucous membranes of the urethra, anus, vagina, and oral cavity. Squamous cells on the cervix can also be involved as can the transitional epithelium of the urethra. Warts are most commonly located over areas that receive friction during coitus and therefore are found near the posterior fourchette of the vulva in women and around the corona of the penis in men. Oral HPV lesions are not common, but can be found in women with external genital warts.

The differential diagnosis for genital warts in women includes vestibular papillomatosis or micropapillomatosis labialis. These are congenital papillations that fill the vestibule with symmetric, smooth-contoured projections. One single projection arises from a base. In contrast, condyloma acuminata have multiple projections from one base and vary in size and distribution. The projections with vestibular papillomatosis may turn white after the application of acetic acid, but that observation does not confirm HPV infection, because there are many other causes of acetowhitening, including acute candidal infection, contact dermatosis, etc. In men, pearly penile papules that are found circumferentially around the tip of the penis may be misdiagnosed as HPV-related external genital warts. These normal papules are symmetrical and are located just under the corona and either side of the adjacent frenulum.

Other lesions that are in the differential diagnosis for the lesions caused by HPV include sebaceous cysts, molluscum contagiosum (especially in HIV-infected patients), and rudimentary hair shafts on the penis. For flat lesions, the differential diagnosis includes vulvar epithelial neoplasia, vaginal intraepithelial neoplasia, and cervical intraepithelial neoplasia depending on location. Condyloma lata, other dermopathies, and invasive carcinoma must also be considered.

Diagnosis

Genital warts are commonly diagnosed by clinical examination. They may appear as typical peaked, cauliflower-like lesions; smooth papules; papules with a rough, horny layer; or as flat lesions. Testing for HPV is not useful in either the clinical diagnosis or the management of external genital warts. HPV testing for high risk types is only clinically useful for women being screened for cervical cancer. Further treatment guidelines for abnormal cervical cytology and histology results can be found through the American Society for Colposcopy and Cervical Pathology [24].

Biopsy of a suspicious lesion should be performed and sent for pathological analysis. Lesions are considered suspicious when they are surrounded by thickened skin, pigmentation, or unexplained ulcerations; raised, bleeding, red, or pigmented; indurated, fixed, or large (>2 cm); unresponsive to targeted therapy; and whenever a suspicion for malignancy exists. Warts in hosts who are immunocompromised

(HIV-infected) and/or who are at risk for HPV-related malignancy (chronic warts, heaving smoking) should also be biopsied. Biopsy is also indicated if the diagnosis is uncertain. Examination of other areas susceptible to infection is also necessary.

Treatment of Genital Warts

Because warts can be disfiguring and prone to superinfection, treatment is generally recommended. However, it must be recognized that about 20–30 % of patients with genital warts will spontaneously clear the warts. In another 60 % of individuals, localized destruction of the wart will recruit host defenses and clear the HPV infection.

The goal of treatment is clearance of visible warts. Some studies show that treatment may reduce infectivity, but there is no evidence that treatment of warts reduces the risk for cancer or eliminates the virus [25]. Therapies can be used alone or in combination. Mechanical and chemical therapies can debulk large lesions and expose the virus to the immune system and prompt host response. Therapies that directly stimulate the local immune system are also available. An important part of all therapies is the patient education and counseling. HPV infection raises all the relevant questions generally associated with STIs, but adds concerns about potential long-term risks for cancer [26].

The CDC treatment guidelines separate the treatments for genital warts into two general categories: treatments that are patient-applied and those that are provider-administered. Factors that may influence selection of treatment include wart size, wart number, anatomic site of wart, wart morphology, patient preference, as well as cost of treatment, convenience, adverse effects, and provider experience [25–29].

It should be noted that warts on moist skin surfaces or intertriginous folds will usually respond to all treatments better than warts found on dry, keratinized skin [25]. Selection of a treatment modality should recognize that warts found on the keratinized skin of the circumcised penis or labia majora will probably require more treatment sessions than those found under the foreskin of the penis or on the inner folds of the labia minora. Most genital warts will respond within 3 months of treatment regardless of treatment modality chosen [25].

Patient-Applied Therapies

Imiquimod 5 % Cream

Imiquimod is a topical cell-mediated immune response modifier that is recommended for treatment of external genital warts. The patient is instructed to apply a thin layer of cream to visible genital warts 3 times (alternating nights) per week at bedtime. It should be washed off 6–10 h after application [25]. Imiquimod is provided in single use foil packets that can be used for up to 4 months as long as continued improvement is noted. For well-keratinized lesions, softening the surface of the wart by bathing and then disrupting it with vigorous drying with a towel has been suggested just before application. Imiquimod has a petroleum base and theoretically can weaken latex condoms or diaphragms. At any rate, sexual contact is not recommended when the cream is on the skin. Virtually all patients using the cream will develop localized erythema; however, only a small minority (10–15 %) has accompanying pain. The people who do experience pain can be advised to take brief holidays from the drug.

Imiquimod acts as a local immune modulator. It induces local interferon and cytokine release, which triggers both the innate and cell-mediated immune response systems [30, 31]. Complete clearance of warts occurs in 72–84 % of women with use of imiquimod but complete clearance rates in men are only half those seen in women [32]. However, many patients who do not completely clear all their lesions will have a substantial reduction in the numbers and size of remaining lesions. In clinical trials, 81 % of subjects had at least a 50 % reduction in wart area [31]. HPV recurrence rates after treatment with Imiquimod appear to be lower (5–19 %) than with other self-administered treatments [22]. Imiquimod is FDA pregnancy category C.

Podofilox 0.5 % Solution or Gel

Podofilox contains purified extract of podophyllin and is recommended for the treatment of external genital warts not involving mucosal epithelium. The solution should be applied to the lesion with a cotton swab; the gel should be applied with a finger. To avoid irritation, the patient should allow the medication to dry after application before ambulating. Podofilox is applied to visible warts 2 times per day for 3 consecutive days, followed by 4 days of no therapy. This cycle may be repeated up to four cycles, as needed to clear warts. The total wart area treated at any application should not exceed 10 cm^2 and the total volume of podofilox applied should be limited to 0.5 mL per day. The mechanism of action of podofilox is to disrupt cell division. It arrests the formation of the mitotic spindle in metaphase and prevents cell duplication. It may also induce damage in local blood vessels and induce immune response by releasing interleukins. The safety of podophyllin during pregnancy has not been established [25]. Podofilox is currently listed as pregnancy category C.

Sinecatechin Ointment 15 %

Sinecatechin ointment is a green-tea extract that was recently approved for the treatment of external anogenital warts. The mechanism of action is not well understood but probably related to green tea's antioxidative properties as well as potential antiviral and antitumor effects [33]. The ointment is applied to the area with a finger in a thin layer daily and not washed off. It can be used until complete clearance of the wart, but for no longer than 16 weeks. Most common side effects are erythema, pruritis/burning, pain, ulceration, edema, induration, and vesicular rash and the ointment may weaken condoms and diaphragms [25]. In clinical trials, complete clearance of warts was obtained in up to 60 % of patients and recurrence rates were very low, 5–8 % [34–37]. Sinecatechin ointment has yet to be studied in comparison to the other patient applied therapies. It is not recommended for HIV-infected patients, immunocompromised patients including those with HIV, or those with clinical genital herpes as the safety and efficacy has not been established [25]. Safety in pregnancy has also not been established and it is currently listed as pregnancy category C.

Provider-Applied Therapies

Trichloroacetic Acid (TCA) 80–90 % or Bichloracetic Acid (BCA) 80–90 %

These acids coagulate the proteins within the wart and act as chemical cautery. They can be used for the treatment of warts on keratinized and mucosal epithelia. TCA or BCA is recommended for the treatment of external genital warts, vaginal warts, and anal warts. A small amount of TCA or BCA is applied directly to visible warts and is allowed to dry. With treatment, the wart will immediately develop a white "frosting" color. Over the ensuing days to weeks, if successful, the wart will detach and leave an ulcer behind. This may be painful and must be monitored for infection. These complications limit the number of warts treated at a single session.

To ensure accurate placement of the acid on the wart, the blunt end of a wooden cotton-tipped applicator or a urethral swab can be used. If a very small area is to be treated, the wooden stick of a cotton-tipped applicator can be broken to reveal a pointed end. Building a moat of lidocaine ointment around the lesion prevents seepage into the surrounding area and provides some comfort. Other health care providers suggest that applying a small amount of lubricating jelly to the treated warts after treatment with TCA or BCA may contribute to patient comfort.

Care must be taken to avoid contamination of the clean bottle of TCA or BCA by using a new applicator stick each time, therefore an adequate supply of applicators of choice should be readily available. If excessive acid is applied to the patient, the health care provider can use either some talc, sodium bicarbonate (i.e., baking soda), or liquid soap to remove excessive acid [25]. This must be applied immediately because the acid will cause burns in a matter of seconds. Therefore, access to these basic substances should be readily available.

In addition, because TCA and BCA are highly caustic agents they must be stored in an area away from children's reach. Containers of TCA and BCA must also be properly labeled, and all staff working with this substance must be properly educated to avoid confusing these highly caustic agents with acetic acid (vinegar).

Clearance rates of up to 80 % can be expected, but multiple applications at weekly intervals may be made. TCA and BCA are not absorbed into systemic circulation and are safe to use during pregnancy.

Podophyllin Resin 10–25 % Sodium

This chemical is compounded in a tincture of benzoin that is cytotoxic and antimitotic and induces tissue necrosis. Podophyllin is recommended for the treatment of external genital warts and urethral meatus warts. A small amount of the solution is applied to each wart on the external genital and allowed to air-dry to prevent irritation. Treatment can be repeated weekly as needed. Podophyllin is neurotropic; it should not be applied to mucosal surfaces from which it might be systemically absorbed. Moreover, application must be limited to less than 0.5 mL or an area of less than 10 cm^2 of warts per session [25]. Some specialists recommend it be washed off 1–6 h after application to reduce the chance of a local irritation and inflammation. Podophyllin should not be applied to the cervix, vagina, oral cavity, or anal canal. The safety of podophyllin during pregnancy has not been established.

Cryotherapy

Cryotherapy freezes the water within the mitochondria of the cell and causes thermally induced cytolysis. Clinicians can use liquid nitrogen (applied by cotton-tip applicator or spray) or nitrous oxide applied by cryoprobes. Regardless of the device used to deliver the cryotherapy to the lesion, application to the wart should continue until the ice ball has extended approximately 2 mm from the edge of the wart. The lesion is then allowed to thaw. Many providers have found that a second freeze session improves efficacy. It has been shown that the tissue destruction occurs during the thawing portion of this process, so adequate time must be given between the freeze–thaw sessions [28]. Cryotherapy is safe to use during pregnancy.

Liquid nitrogen is recommended for the treatment of external genital warts, vaginal warts, urethral meatal warts, anal warts, and oral warts. If the liquid nitrogen is obtained from a large metal tank, it evaporates quickly; a large portion of the expense comes from frequent refilling of this large tank. A metal ladle is supplied, which is used to fill either the sealed spray canister or Styrofoam cup. Care must be taken when ladling the liquid nitrogen and protective hand coverings should be worn at all times to protect the exposed skin of the health care provider. A Styrofoam cup is used because of its excellent insulation properties; other materials are not as reliable. Regular cotton-tipped applicator sticks are used to apply the liquid nitrogen to the genital wart. Depending on the size of the lesion, it may be useful to form the cotton tip into a point before dipping it into the nitrogen.

When the nitrogen spray canister is used, it is important that the health care provider have excellent hand–eye coordination so that a steady stream of liquid nitrogen is directed at the lesion only, sparing unaffected surrounding tissue. This will take practice to become proficient, especially when treating small warts.

Nitrogen also comes as compressed gas form (nitrous oxide), which is attached to a cryoprobe with a tip that matches the size and shape of the wart. This is the same handheld cryoprobe used to treat cervical dysplasia. Gaseous nitrogen is recommended for the treatment of external genital warts. A small amount of lubricating jelly may be applied to the cryoprobe or to the genital wart to help transfer the cold to the lesion. The trigger is pulled back, allowing the refrigerant to enter the gun, which freezes the tip and the jelly covering the wart. Because the freezing is more intense and less controlled with the cryoprobe, it is not recommended for use in cryotherapy of lesions on their mucosal surfaces such as the urethra or vagina.

Overall, clearance rates with cryotherapy are up to 90 %, recurrence rates approach 40 % [38].

Surgical Therapies

In general, this therapy is reserved for large or medium lesions and those that are unresponsive to medical therapies. The warts are removed at the dermal–epidermal junction. Various techniques that can be used in different settings include scissor excision, shave excision, curettage, LEEP, electrocautery, and laser. Treatment may lead to scarring and vulvodynia if too deep a removal is performed, especially with LEEP. Often surgical excision is done under local anesthesia and requires specialist training.

However, surgical excision can be easily performed in the office to remove a wart that is pedunculated on a slender (1–2 mm) stalk. This type of wart is quite commonly seen in perianal area. After cleaning the area, lift the wart, visualize the separation line between the epidermis and the wart and cut across the base of the lesion along that line. Hemostasis is generally easily obtained by pressure and the use of Monsel solution or other chemical styptic.

Carbon dioxide laser therapy may be useful for extensive vulvar warts and anal warts, especially if other therapies have failed. It is also the preferred treatment for immunocompromised, nonpregnant patients with large lesions. All the lesions may be destroyed in one treatment, although healing may be uncomfortable. Laser therapy has been associated long-term with vulvodynia, particularly if the deeper tissue layers are burned. Recurrence rates are low in the immediate posttreatment period.

Alternative Therapies

The CDC treatment guidelines also offer a few alternative regimens including intralesional interferon, photodynamic therapy, and topical cidofovir. These regimens are considered alternates as they may cause more side effects or have limited efficacy data [25, 26].

Combination Therapies

The CDC treatment guidelines note that because each of the available treatments has shortcomings, some clinics employ combination therapy (i.e., the simultaneous use of two or more modalities on the same wart at the same time) [25]. As data is limited on the efficacy and risk of this practice, clinicians may want to use different treatment modalities sequentially. For example, a clinician may start therapy with TCA and have the patient return later for cryotherapy to remove persistent lesions. In another approach, at least one study has demonstrated the efficacy of up to 16 weeks of treatment with imiquimod followed by surgical removal of any remaining genital warts; recurrence rates were also reduced [39].

Patient Education and Counseling

The psychological impact of diagnosis of HPV infection may be even more profound than that of other STIs. In addition to issues of relationship fidelity, there is the issue of oncogenic potential, which requires additional counseling [40].

College-aged women are at particularly high risk for acquiring HPV infection. The diagnosis can cause confusion and distress for women; they may need psychological support and information from their health care provider. Patients with HPV on pap smears report that the diagnosis created a negative effect on their sexual contact and on their relationship with their partner [41, 42]. One large study of patients with HPV found that a majority rated their provider as fair or poor in counseling them [43]. Patients were most disturbed by the lack of advice about emotional issues. Survey of clinicians in college-based clinics recognized the patient's need for information but 46 % spent less than 10 min providing education and counseling to newly diagnosed patients [40].

Patients often may ask how long the infection has been there and when and where was the infection acquired. It is not possible for the clinician to answer these questions accurately. The HPV infection may be subclinical (without visible lesions) for many months or years. A period of decreased immunity (as seen in pregnancy) or increased stress may trigger the growth of warts. It is important for the patient to understand three other points:

- Genital HPV infection is common among sexually active adults.
- Genital HPV infection is usually sexually transmitted, but the sex partner probably is not aware that infection is present.
- HPV testing is not warranted for the patient or the partner.

Follow-up

Follow-up at 3 months can be offered to patients who have cleared anogenital warts. This will provide an opportunity to evaluate for recurrent warts and to continue to provide patient education. Female patients who have had a history of anogenital warts should be advised to receive annual pap smears to evaluate for cervical abnormalities. Self-examination for external genital warts may be encouraged.

Partner Notification and Reporting Requirements

There is no legal requirement to notify sexual contacts. It is known that most sex partners of individuals infected with HPV are themselves infected. There is no documented evidence that professional examination of sex partners is necessary. Treatment of the partner has not been shown to reduce the patient's risk for recurrence. Recurrence of anogenital warts can result from reactivation of a latent infection. For these reasons, the CDC treatment guidelines do not mandate partner notification or treatment in the absence of grossly visible lesions. However, it should be noted that a visit to a health care provider affords an excellent opportunity to provide education and to screen for other STIs in all patients. Female partners of men with external genital warts should be encouraged to receive routine pap smears [25].

Pregnancy-Related Issues

During pregnancy, HPV tends be expressed or reactivated, potentially due to a pregnant woman's relative immune system suppression. This does not necessarily mean a recent inoculation/infection with HPV, but probably represents a latent infection or a reactivation of an old infection. The incidence of laryngeal papillomatosis in infants and children is extremely rare and the mechanism of transmission is not entirely understood. Despite the possibility of vertical transmission, vaginal delivery is the preferred method of delivery for women with genital warts. However, occasionally, a cesarean section will be recommended when extensive lesions obstruct the outlet of the birth canal or they create a concern that laceration/episiotomy repair would not be possible [25]. Treatment of external genital warts during pregnancy is generally advocated because the lesions tend to grow in the immunocompromised state and may become superinfected although wart resolution may be incomplete. Imiquimod, sinecatechins, podophyllin, and podofilox should not be used and tiny asymptomatic lesions may not warrant treatment.

HIV-Related Issues

People infected with HPV are both more likely to develop genital warts and to have more difficult-to-treat warts than people without HIV. While there is no data to suggest specific treatment modalities for the HIV-infected patient, it should be noted that they might not respond as well to therapy or be prone to more frequent wart recurrences [25].

Prevention

There are currently two HPV vaccines licensed for use in the United States: a quadrivalent vaccine (Gardasil) and a bivalent vaccine (Cervarix). Both vaccines provide protection against HPV 16 and 18, responsible for about two thirds of all cervical cancers while Gardasil also targets HPV types 6 and 11 found in nearly 90 % of anogenital warts. Both vaccines are given in a 3 dose series at 0, 2, and 6 months. Either can be given to girls aged 9–26 [44, 45] while the quadravalent vaccine can also be used in boys 9–26 years old to prevent genital warts [46]. Vaccinated women not previously exposed to these HPV types are expected to have a 90 % reduction in genital infection from those HPV types [47–49].

The vaccines should ideally be administered before the onset of sexual activity but should still be offered after sexual debut. Furthermore, women who have received HPV vaccination should continue routine cervical cancer screening as HPV types 16 and 18 account for only 70 % of cervical cancers.

Avoiding skin-to-skin contact with an infected partner is the most effective approach to prevent HPV infection. Condom use has been shown to protect against the acquisition of genital HPV infection. A study of newly sexually active college women showed a 70 % risk reduction in HPV transmission with correct and consistent condom use [50]. Furthermore, condom use reduces HPV-related diseases, such as genital warts in men and cervical dysplasia in women and is associated with higher rates of regression of these conditions [13, 51].

References

1. The Henry J. Kaiser Family Foundation. Fact sheet: sexually transmitted diseases in the U.S. Available from: http://www.kff.org/womenshealth/1447-std_fs.cfm. Accessed 31 Dec 2012.
2. Gerberding JL. Report to congress: prevention of genital human papillomavirus infection. Atlanta, GA: Centers for Disease Control and Prevention, Department of Health and Human Services; 2004.
3. The Centers for Disease Control and Prevention. 2011 Sexually transmitted diseases surveillance table; 2011. Available from: http://www.cdc.gov/std/stats11/tables/44.htm. Accessed 31 Dec 2012.

4. Cates Jr W. Estimates of the incidence and prevalence of sexually transmitted diseases in the United States. American Social Health Association Panel. Sex Transm Dis. 1999;26:S2–7.
5. Myers ER, McCrory DC, Nanda K, Bastian L, Matchar DB. Mathematical model for the natural history of human papillomavirus infection and cervical carcinogenesis. Am J Epidemiol. 2000;151:1158–71.
6. Weinstock H, Berman S, Cates Jr W. Sexually transmitted diseases among American youth: incidence and prevalence estimates, 2000. Perspect Sex Reprod Health. 2004;36:6–10.
7. Ho GY, Bierman R, Beardsley L, Chang CJ, Burk RD. Natural history of cervicovaginal papillomavirus infection in young women. N Engl J Med. 1998;338:423–8.
8. Silins I, Kallings I, Dillner J. Correlates of the spread of human papillomavirus infection. Cancer Epidemiol Biomarkers Prev. 2000;9:953–9.
9. Sellors JW, Mahony JB, Kaczorowski J, et al. Prevalence and predictors of human papillomavirus infection in women in Ontario, Canada. Survey of HPV in Ontario Women (SHOW) Group. CMAJ. 2000;163:503–8.
10. Sellors JW, Karwalajtys TL, Kaczorowski J, et al. Incidence, clearance and predictors of human papillomavirus infection in women. CMAJ. 2003;168:421–5.
11. Bauer HM, Hildesheim A, Schiffman MH, et al. Determinants of genital human papillomavirus infection in low-risk women in Portland, Oregon. Sex Transm Dis. 1993;20:274–8.
12. Munoz N, Bosch FX, de Sanjose S, et al. Epidemiologic classification of human papillomavirus types associated with cervical cancer. N Engl J Med. 2003;348:518–27.
13. Bleeker MC, Hogewoning CJ, Voorhorst FJ, et al. Condom use promotes regression of human papillomavirus-associated penile lesions in male sexual partners of women with cervical intraepithelial neoplasia. Int J Cancer. 2003;107:804–10.
14. Marrazzo JM, Koutsky LA, Stine KL, et al. Genital human papillomavirus infection in women who have sex with women. J Infect Dis. 1998;178:1604–9.
15. Cox T, Buck HW, Kinney W, Rubin MM. HPV types: natural history and epidemiology. Human papillomavirus (HPV) and cervical cancer. Clinical proceedings. Washington, DC: Association of Reproductive Health Professionals; 2001. Available from: org/healthcareproviders/onlinepublications/clinicalproceedings/cphpv/types.cfm?ID=149. Accessed 24 Nov 2006.
16. Mao C, Hughes JP, Kiviat N, et al. Clinical findings among young women with genital human papillomavirus infection. Am J Obstet Gynecol. 2003;188:677–84.
17. Perniciaro C, Dicken CH. Tanning bed warts. J Am Acad Dermatol. 1988;18:586–7.
18. Blackledge FA, Anand VK. Tracheobronchial extension of recurrent respiratory papillomatosis. Ann Otol Rhinol Laryngol. 2000;109:812–8.
19. Silverberg MJ, Thorsen P, Lindeberg H, Grant LA, Shah KV. Condyloma in pregnancy is strongly predictive of juvenile-onset recurrent respiratory papillomatosis. Obstet Gynecol. 2003;101:645–52.
20. Byars RW, Poole GV, Barber WH. Anal carcinoma arising from condyloma acuminata. Am Surg. 2001;67:469–72.
21. Rubin MA, Kleter B, Zhou M, et al. Detection and typing of human papillomavirus DNA in penile carcinoma: evidence for multiple independent pathways of penile carcinogenesis. Am J Pathol. 2001;159:1211–8.
22. Gunter J. Genital and perianal warts: new treatment opportunities for human papillomavirus infection. Am J Obstet Gynecol. 2003;189:S3–11.
23. Arany I, Evans T, Tyring SK. Tissue specific HPV expression and downregulation of local immune responses in condylomas from HIV seropositive individuals. Sex Transm Infect. 1998;74:349–53.
24. American Society for Colposcopy and Cervical Pathology. Consensus guidelines: cytology algorithms and HPV genotyping algorithm. Available from: http://www.asccp.org. Accessed 5 Jan 2013.
25. Centers for Disease Control and Prevention. Sexually transmitted diseases treatment guidelines 2010. Available from: http://www.cdc.gov/std/treatment/2010/genital-warts.htm. Accessed 31 Dec 2012.

26. Lacey CJ. Therapy for genital human papillovirus-related disease. J Clin Virol. 2005;32 Suppl 1:S82–90.
27. Langley PC, Richwald GA, Smith MH. Modeling the impact of treatment options in genital warts: patient-applied versus physician-administered therapies. Clin Ther. 1999;21:2143–55.
28. Kodner CM, Nasraty S. Management of genital warts. Am Fam Physician. 2004;70:2335–42.
29. Lacey CJ, Goodall RL, Tennvall GR, et al. Randomized controlled trial and economic evaluation of podophyllotoxin solution, podophyllotoxin cream, and podophyllin in the treatment of genital warts. Sex Transm Infect. 2003;79:270–5.
30. Dahl MV. Imiquimod: an immune response modifier. J Am Acad Dermatol. 2000;43:S1–5.
31. Tyring SK, Arany I, Stanley MA, et al. A randomized, controlled, molecular study of condylomata acuminata clearance during treatment with imiquimod. J Infect Dis. 1998;178:551–5.
32. Edwards L, Ferenczy A, Eron L, et al. Self-administered topical 5% imiquimod cream for external anogenital warts. Arch Dermatol. 1998;134:25–30.
33. Melzer SM, Monk BJ, Tewari KS. Green tea catechins for treatment of external genital warts. Am J Obstet Gynecol. 2009;200:233.e1–e7.
34. Tatti S, Swinehart JM, Thielert C, et al. Sinecatechins, a defined green tea extract, in the treatment of external anogenital warts: a randomized controlled trial. Obstet Gynecol. 2008;111:1371–9.
35. Tzellos TG, Sardelli C, Lallas A, et al. Efficacy, safety and tolerability of green tea catechins in the treatment of external anogenital warts: a systematic review and meta-analysis. J Eur Acad Dermatol Venereol. 2011;25(3):345–53.
36. Stockfleth E, Beti H, Orasan R, et al. Topical Polyphenon E in the treatment of external genital and perianal warts: a randomized controlled trial. Br J Dermatol. 2008;158:1329–38.
37. Gross G, Meyer KG, Pres H, et al. A randomized, double-blind, four-arm parallel-group, placebo-controlled phase II/III study to investigate the clinical efficacy of two galenic formulations of Polyphenon E in the treatment of external genital warts. J Eur Acad Dermatol Venereol. 2007;21:1404–12.
38. Maw RD. Treatment of anogenital warts. Dermatol Clin. 1998;16:829–34.
39. Carrasco D, vander Straten M, Tyring SK. Treatment of anogenital warts with imiquimod 5% cream followed by surgical excision of residual lesions. J Am Acad Dermatol. 2002;47:S212–6.
40. Linnehan MJ, Groce NE. Psychosocial and educational services for female college students with genital human papillomavirus infection. Fam Plann Perspect. 1999;31:137–41.
41. Campion MJ, Brown JR, McCance DJ, et al. Psychosexual trauma of an abnormal cervical smear. Br J Obstet Gynaecol. 1988;95:175–81.
42. Filiberti A, Tamburini M, Stefanon B, et al. Psychological aspects of genital human papillomavirus infection: a preliminary report. J Psychosom Obstet Gynecol. 1993;14:145–52.
43. Guy H. Survey shows how we live with HPV. HPV News. 1993;3(1):4–8.
44. CDC. Quadrivalent human papillomavirus vaccine: recommendations of the Advisory Committee on Immunization Practices (ACIP). Morb Mortal Wkly Rep. 2007;56(No. RR-2):1–24.
45. CDC. FDA licensure of bivalent human papillomavirus vaccine (HPV2, Cervarix) for use in females and updated HPV vaccination recommendations from the Advisory Committee on Immunization Practices (ACIP). Morb Mortal Wkly Rep. 2010;59:626–9.
46. CDC. FDA licensure of quadrivalent human papillomavirus vaccine (HPV4, Gardasil) for use in males and guidance from the Advisory Committee on Immunization Practices (ACIP). Morb Mortal Wkly Rep. 2010;59:630–2.
47. Koutsky LA, Ault KA, Wheeler CM, et al. A controlled trial of a human papillomavirus type 16 vaccine. N Engl J Med. 2002;347:1645–51.
48. Harper DM, Franco EL, Wheeler C, et al. Efficacy of a bivalent L1 virus-like particle vaccine in prevention of infection with human papillomavirus types 16 and 18 in young women: a randomised controlled trial. Lancet. 2004;364:1757–65.

49. Villa LL, Costa RL, Petta CA, et al. Prophylactic quadrivalent human papillomavirus (types 6, 11, 16, and 18) L1 virus-like particle vaccine in young women: a randomised double-blind placebo-controlled multicentre phase II efficacy trial. Lancet Oncol. 2005;6:271–8.
50. Winer RL, Hughes JP, Feng Q, et al. Condom use and the risk of genital human papillomavirus infection in young women. N Engl J Med. 2006;354:2645–54.
51. Hogewoning CJ, Bleeker MC, van den Brule AJ, et al. Condom use promotes regression of cervical intraepithelial neoplasia and clearance of human papillomavirus: a randomized clinical trial. Int J Cancer. 2003;107:811–6.

Chapter 2
Genital Herpes

D. Gene Parks

Introduction

Herpes simplex virus (HSV) has a long and confusing history. More than 2,500 years ago, Hippocrates first used the word "herpes," derived from the Greek word "to creep," to describe how the lesions of this contagious ulcerative disease seemed to creep or crawl along the skin [1]. Galen first noted that recurrences develop at the same anatomic site. However, over time, the word herpes was used to describe many skin conditions from lupus to zoster. The definition of herpes (particularly oral lesions) became more rigorous in the seventeenth century. In the 1830s, recurrent genital herpes was described and 60 years later was identified as a "vocational disease"—a sexually transmitted infection (STI). The virus itself was not identified until the 1950s. In 1971, it was proposed that two different types of HSV caused infection. HSV-1 commonly causes labial or pharyngeal infection, and transmission is primary by nongenital contact. HSV-2 typically affects the genital area and is transmitted by intimate sexual contact. However, both viruses are capable of causing either genital or oral-pharyngeal infections that appear identical on examination. In the United States, HSV infection is one of the most common STIs and is the leading cause of genital ulcers.

Fast Facts

- Genital herpes is one of the most prevalent STIs in the United States. About 50 million Americans have genital HSV infection.

D.G. Parks, MD (✉)

Department of Obstetrics and Gynecology, David Geffen School of Medicine at UCLA, 4560 Admiralty Way #303, Marina Del Rey, Los Angeles, CA 90292, USA
e-mail: Drgeneparks@aol.com

N.S. Skolnik et al. (eds.), *Sexually Transmitted Diseases: A Practical Guide for Primary Care*, Current Clinical Practice, DOI 10.1007/978-1-62703-499-9_2,
© Springer Science+Business Media New York 2013

- HSV is the leading cause of genital ulcers. HSV-2 infections at least doubles the risk of sexual acquisition of human immunodeficiency virus (HIV) and also increases transmission.
- Herpes is a chronic, lifelong infection; patients can shed virus, not only during outbreaks but also during asymptomatic periods.
- Intrapartum transmission of HSV-2 can cause neonatal death or permanent neurological damage.
- Testing for HSV-2 antibodies is not recommended for general population screening.

Prevalence and Incidence

The full extent of the HSV epidemic in the United States is not known because (1) HSV infection is not a reportable disease in most states, (2) most people carrying the virus are not aware that they are infected, and (3) it is not possible in many cases for people to distinguish between an initial outbreak (incidence) and a recurrence (prevalence).

Serology studies suggest that 50 million people in the United States have genital HSV infection. In Europe, HSV-2 is found in 8–15 % of the general population. In Africa, the prevalence rates are 40–50 % in 20-year-olds. Between the two most recent iterations of National Health and Nutritional Examination Surveys (NHANES)—NHANES in 1988–1994 and NHANES in 1999–2004—the seroprevalence of HSV-2 among civilian, noninstitutionalized people aged 14–49 in the United States decreased by 19 % from 21 to 17 % [2]. By contrast, 57.7 % of the same group was seropositive for HSV-1 in 1999–2004, which represents a 6.9 % decline. Seroprevalence for HSV-2 increases with age, being virtually nonexistent in children under age 12, and stabilizing after age 30; this pattern is consistent with the virus being an STI. By contrast, HSV-1 seroprevalence in children under 5 is 20 % and rises in a linear fashion until age 20. This pattern is not characteristic of an STI. More than 85 % of the world's adult population is seropositive for HSV-1.

The NHANES surveys found that women (23.1 %) are more likely to be seropositive than men (11.2 %). Seropositivity is highest among blacks (40.3 %), followed by whites (13.7 %) and Hispanics (11.9 %). Lifetime numbers of sex partners influenced seropositivity, varying from 2.6 % of patients with no sex partners to 39.9 %, for people with at least 50 partners [2]. Patient history is very unreliable for obtaining information about this infection.

Of the 50 million Americans who are HSV seropositive, only 9 % is aware of having had a previous infection [3]. Even when seropositive individuals are asked specific questions, only 25–33 % admits having had symptoms consistent with genital herpes. Approximately 75 % of source partners discover their own infection only when their newly infected partner is diagnosed [4].

It is estimated that there are 1.6 million new cases of genital HSV infections in the United States each year [5], and 10 million recurrences annually [6]. Worldwide, 20 million new people are infected each year [7].

Herpes infections are troubling enough by themselves, but they also represent a risk factor for acquiring and spreading other STIs. Herpes is one of the most common infections found in HIV-infected adults; 90 % of HIV patients are also infected with HSV (see Chap. 4). Several studies have established a causative relationship between HSV genital ulcerations and HIV acquisition, transmission, and progression [8]. High titers of HIV are found in genital herpes ulcerations [9]. In addition, HIV infection reactivation is accompanied by an increase in plasma HIV viral load [10]. A meta-analysis of studies that documented HSV-2 infection before HIV acquisition found that the HSV more than doubled the risk; the relative risk was 2.1 (95 %, CI: 1.4–3.2). About 52 % of HIV infection is attributable to HSV-2 coinfection. The population attributable risk percentage varied with HSV-2 prevalence and ranged from 19 to 47 % [11].

Risk Factors

HSV-2 infects all economic classes, race, ages, and ethnic groups. However, there are identifiable risk factors for HSV-2 infection, which reflect biological and behavioral influences. Major risk factors for seropositivity include female gender, ethnicity (African-American or Hispanic), history of STIs, increasing number of sex partners, sexual contact with commercial sex workers, cocaine use, and low socioeconomic status or level of education. In addition, older age and young age at sexual debut are important factors [12]. Each additional sex act per week increases the risk of acquiring genital herpes [13]. In a study of discordant monogamous couples, risk factors for HSV acquisition were female gender and the absence of HSV-1 antibodies [4]. Other risk factors that have been shown to be independent predictors of HSV-2 infection in women include cigarette smoking, douching, history of having intercourse with an uncircumcised male partner, the presence of vaginal group B streptococcus, and abnormal vaginal flora [14].

Infectivity and Transmission

Herpes is highly contagious. In a study of newly acquired HSV infections the median number of sex acts before transmission was 40 [45]. Seventy-five percent of sexual partners of HSV-2-infected people contract the disease. In a study of seronegative sexually active individuals, the annual rates of infection were 1.6 % for HSV-1 and 5.1 % for HSV-2 [15]; the primary route of transmission of HSV-2 infection is genital-to-genital skin contact with an infected partner who is shedding virus symptomatically or asymptomatically. HSV-2 is responsible for about 80 % of genital herpes infections, even though there are as many initial cases with HSV-1 infection, which is usually acquired through oral–genital contact, HSV-2 is more likely to cause recurrent episodes. HSV-1 genital infections are higher in men who have sex with men (MSM) [16].

Asymptomatic shedding is responsible for most of the transmission of HSV [4, 17]. HSV DNA has been detected by polymerase chain reaction (PCR) from genital samples of HSV-2-infected women on 28 % of days [18]. In discordant couples, 69 % of transmission occurred when the infected partner was asymptomatic [4]. Transmission of HSV between discordant sexual partners occurs at a rate of about 10 % per year [19]. Asymptomatic shedding is more common with HSV-2 than with HSV-1 infection [20].

Although transmission of HSV infections generally results from intimate skin-to-skin contact with an infected individual, it can also result from exposure to infected saliva, semen, vaginal secretions, or fluid from active herpetic lesions.

Drying and room temperature quickly inactivate the virus. Therefore, HSV transmission is not believed to occur often through exposure to fomites.

Etiology

HSV belongs to the Herpesviridae family, which also includes the cytomegalovirus, Epstein–Barr virus, and varicella-zoster virus. HSV-1 and HSV-2 are two of the eight human herpes viruses; neither is found in other animal species.

HSV is an enveloped, double-stranded DNA virus. HSV-1 and HSV-2 are distinguished by antigenic differences in their envelope proteins [4]. However, the genomes of the two viruses are 50 % homologous. There are multiple specific strains of HSV-1 and HSV-2.

After contact with abraded skin or mucosal surfaces, the virus replicates and initiates infection in the epidermal cells of the target area. Following this initial infection, the virus travels in a retrograde fashion within axons of sensory nerves to the dorsal nerve root ganglion where it continues to replicate to establish lifelong latency [3]. HSV-2 usually migrates to the sacral nerve roots (S2, S3, and S4). Recurrent outbreaks localized to the dermatomes innervated by the infected nerve are quite common, especially with HSV-2. In patients with an initial primary episode of genital herpes, the risk of having at least one recurrence during the first year is nearly 90 % [21]. Although some HSV-2-infected patients may not experience symptomatic recurrences, virtually all will have repeated episodes of asymptomatic viral shedding from their genital secretions. This shedding places their sexual contacts at risk for acquiring the infection.

Clinical Manifestations

There are three types of HSV genital infections: primary infection, non-primary initial infection, and recurrent infection (see Table 2.1). A primary infection is the first HSV infection that occurs in a patient without prior exposure to HSV, as demonstrated by the fact that the patient has no antibodies to HSV. An initial,

Table 2.1 Definition of genital herpes syndromes

Initial primary infection
Initial infection with either herpes type 1 or herpes type 2 in a patient who has had no prior exposure to either HSV-1 or HSV-2 (seronegative for HSV-1 and HSV-2)
Initial non-primary infection
First clinical infection with either HSV-1 or HSV-2 in a patient who has had prior exposure to the other HSV
Recurrent infection
A recurrence, not a reinfection. The infection results from reactivation of a latent virus

Source: Modified from [26], p. 102

HSV herpes simplex virus

non-primary infection is defined as a first HSV infection with one HSV type in a patient who is already infected with another type of HSV (e.g., a new HSV-2 infection in a patient with prior HSV-1 infection). Because HSV-1 is so prevalent, most initial genital infections (usually with HSV-2) are initial, non-primary infections. Recurrent infections are outbreaks owing to reactivation of a previously acquired HSV infection (not a reinfection).

The incubation period after genital exposure to HSV-1 or HSV-2 is approximately 4 days (range 2–12 days) [22]. Almost half of first-episode genital herpes is caused by HSV-1. The local and systemic symptoms with primary genital infections are generally the same intensity and duration for both HSV-1 and HSV-2 [23].

The classical clinical presentation of genital herpes starts with widespread multiple painful macules and papules, which then mature into clusters of clear, fluid-filled vesicles and pustules. The vesicles rupture and form ulcers. Skin ulcers crust, whereas lesions on mucous membranes heal without crusting [22]. Scarring does not usually occur after re-epithelization. Secondary bacterial infections may produce ulcers that extend into the dermis or that cause cellulitis. In women, the ulcers occur at the introitus, labia, perineum, or perianal area. Patients complain of dysuria, vulvar pain, dyspareunia, and increased vaginal discharge and bleeding. Patients may volitionally retain urine because the pain with urination is so severe. On average, initial primary infections last 12 days, but viral shedding continues for 20–21 days [24]. The infection may be spread by autoinoculation to other areas of the genitalia as well as to the buttocks and thighs and to distant sites, such as the conjunctivae. Urethral involvement is common; 82 % of patients with initial infection have urethritis with positive urethral cultures. Cervical infection, which is found in 80 % of women, causes increased vaginal discharge and postcoital spotting and bleeding. Men usually develop lesions on the penile shaft or glands. The patient usually develops tender inguinal adenopathy. Perianal infections are also common in MSM. Pharyngitis may develop with oral exposure.

Initial primary infection is associated with a higher rate of systemic involvement and greater severity of local disease than is seen with initial non-primary genital herpes infection. With primary infections, 66 % of women and 40 % of men develop constitutional symptoms such as fever, malaise, nausea, headache, myalgia, hepatitis, meningitis, and autonomic nervous system dysfunction as a result of viremia [22]. Approximately 30 % of women and 10 % of men have headache, stiff neck, and photophobia with or without fever [22]; 4 % of individuals will develop viral meningitis [25]. The meningitis is transient and requires no treatment; it resolves without any sequelae. Infection in the sacral plexus may affect sensation in the pelvis as well as detrusor function; 10–15 % of women with initial disease will develop urinary retention that requires catheterization. This nerve dysfunction may last 6–7 weeks [3]. HIV-infected individuals are at higher risk of developing the more serious clinical manifestations, including dissemination, encephalitis, and meningoencephalitis [25].

Most initial genital herpes infections are not "classical" in their presentation. The majority of initial infections are asymptomatic or atypical; patients note nonspecific symptoms of discharge, dysuria, pain, erythema, back pain, pruritus, soreness, fissure, and folliculitis and think they have a rash, allergy, yeast infection, cystitis, zipper trauma, jock itch, or bike seat irritation [26]. Clinicians often fail to diagnose HSV infection and attribute the signs and symptoms to other diagnoses, particularly when there are only small blisters or ulcers, vaginal lesions, urethritis or cervicitis without external lesions, excoriation, fissures, or nonspecific erythema [27]. About 1 in 7 men who present with sores, blisters, ulcers, crusting, or small cuts/slits had HSV and about 1 in 9 women with redness, irritation, or rash have HSV [8]. The relative mildness of the symptoms and subtlety of the physical findings may occur because most initial infections with HSV-2 occur in people who carry antibodies to HSV-1. There are generally fewer lesions with these non-primary initial infections. Systemic symptoms develop in only 16 % of people with initial non-primary infections. The duration of infection in this situation is shorter (9 days) and viral shedding lasts only 1 week [28]. Thus, genital herpes infection should be considered routinely in any patient with genital lesions. This would include patients with genital erythema, rash, skin fissuring, pain, burning, or genital itch.

Recurrent infections are more common and occur more frequently with HSV-2 than with HSV-1 infection. Within 1 year of diagnosis of initial primary HSV-2 genital infections, 90 % of people will have at least one recurrence, whereas only 55 % of HSV-1-infected people have repeat outbreaks. In one study, nearly 40 % of the HSV-2-infected subjects had six or more recurrences [21]. Median time to recurrence with HSV-2 was 49 days, whereas median time to recurrence of HSV-1 was 310 days. Most recurrences are asymptomatic. About half of patients who recognize recurrences report prodromal symptoms, such as localized tingling, pruritus, or pain 30 min to 48 h before eruption. Some patients experience more painful and prolonged prodromes including shooting pain in the buttocks, hips, or legs for up to 5 days [22]. Recurrent herpes outbreaks are usually less severe than primary outbreaks. The numbers of lesions are generally fewer. The lesions may appear the same as in primary outbreaks but heal in half the time or they may present as fissures or vulvar erythema rather than typical ulcers. About 10–15 % patients with recurrent genital herpes will have coexisting cervical disease. Systemic manifestations do not occur with recurrences in immunocompetent patients. Over time, recurrence rates decrease [29].

Frequently, women who have HSV-related ulcers become superinfected with Candida. Prompt attention to treating that infection can decrease the patient's discomfort.

Factors other than HSV type that have been associated with frequency of recurrent outbreaks include fatigue, menstruation, intercourse, and trauma. The most common cause of recurrence of HSV in HIV-infected patients is the degree of immunosuppression. Although it is commonly believed that acute episodes of stress are associated with onset of recurrent herpes, studies have concluded that only persistent stress lasting longer than 1 week and depression are psychological stressors that are associated with onset of recurrent outbreaks [3].

Testing Techniques

Until recently, viral isolation in cell culture and determination of the type of HSV with fluorescent staining has been the mainstay of herpes testing in patients presenting with characteristic genital lesions. The cytopathic cell changes induced by the herpes virus in tissue culture usually occurs within 3 days of inoculation but the cell culture is not considered negative for herpes until a final negative reading on day 15. The rate of recovery of the virus depends on the stage of the clinical disease being tested. There is a 90 % chance of obtaining a positive culture when the specimen is obtained from the base of a freshly unroofed vesicle or pustule, but that sensitivity decreases to 70 % when the specimen is obtained from an existing herpes ulcer and drops to only 27 % when a crusted lesion is used as a specimen source. The probability of recovery of the virus from a patient with recurrent herpes, which has a much shorter duration of viral shedding and a lower viral load, is only 30 %.

The Tzanck preparation is a histological examination of lesions that identifies the presence of a DNA virus with multinucleated giant cells typical of HSV. Although the test is rapid, it is not specific for HSV. Similar changes can be found in sites infected with the varicella virus. Similarly, cytological detection of HSV infection (e.g., from pap smear) is not only insensitive, it is nonspecific and has a low positive predictive rate. It should not be used for diagnosis.

PCR assay for HSV DNA has been shown to be more sensitive than viral culture and has a specificity that exceeds 99.9 %. The PCR test is the standard of care test for the diagnosis of herpes central nervous system infection. The PCR is highly accurate and faster than tissue culture. Its use in clinical practice is currently expanding due to its higher sensitivity than traditional tissue cell culture [30].

Commercially available blood tests that can identify prior exposure by testing for HSV-specific glycoproteins G2 (HSV-2) and G1 (HSV-1) immunoglobulin (IgG) G antibodies. These two Food and Drug Administration (FDA)-approved tests for laboratory use are HerpeSelect™-1 enzyme-linked immunosorbent assay (ELISA) IgG, and HerpeSelect 1 and 2 Immunoblot IgG (for HSV-1 and HSV-2) (Focus Diagnostics, Herndon, VA). They have a sensitivity of detecting HSV-2 of 98 % and

Table 2.2 Guidelines for type-specific HSV serological tests

Diagnosis of genital lesions/symptoms: type-specific serology tests should be available for diagnostic purposes in conjunction with virological tests at clinical settings that provide care for patients with STDs or those at risk at risk for STDs. Serology tests may be useful in the following situations
A culture-negative recurrent lesion
A history suggestive of herpes/atypical herpes with no lesions to culture
The first presentation of genital symptoms when culture or antigen detection is negative or not available
Screening for HIV-positive patients should be generally offered
Patients in partnerships or considering partnerships with HSV-2 infected people (especially if it would change behavior)
HIV-infected people may benefit from testing during their first evaluation
Universal screening in pregnancy should not be generally offered
Screening in general population should not be generally offered
Herpes education and prevention counseling is necessary for all people being screened for HSV-2

HSV herpes simplex virus, *STD* sexually transmitted disease, *HIV* human immunodeficiency virus

a specificity of 97–100 % because of their ability to detect glycoprotein G-2 for HSV-2 and glycoproteins G-1 and C-1 for HSV-1. Two point-of-care tests are also available: Biokit HSV-2 and SureVac HSV-2.

The older tests should never be ordered to determine a specific type of herpes. Seroconversion of an initial primary herpes attack will usually occur 12 weeks after the outbreak [30]. Therefore, HSV-2 serological testing cannot detect a primary infection; it can be used only to rule out recurrent infections. The CDC list of appropriate use of serologic testing is summarized in Table 2.2.

Screening in the general population should generally not be offered. More detail of situations in which testing might be appropriate is provided here.

1. Diagnosis of HSV-2

   (a) Patients who present with a 3-month or greater history of recurrent genital lesions suggestive of recurrent genital herpes but have no lesions on exam or have recent negative viral culture for herpes. A negative HSV-1 and HSV-2 serological test would rule out genital herpes as the cause of the lesions, whereas a positive HSV-2 serology would support the diagnosis of recurrent genital herpes. Interpretation of a positive HSV-1 test would be more difficult. However, it must be recognized that the recurrent symptoms may be owing to an unrelated lesion.

   (b) Patients who have first presentation of genital symptoms when culture or antigen detection is negative or not available. Note: testing would have to be delayed by 12 weeks to allow for antibody formulation.

2. HIV-infected patients. Because of the high coinfection rate with HSV, all HIV-infected patients should be offered type-specific HSV serological testing.

3. Partner consideration. The evaluation of patient who is in a partnership or is considering partnership with a person with documented genital herpes and is

concerned about the possible transmission. If the asymptomatic person is HSV-2-seropositive, then the couple can be reassured that further transmission between them cannot take place. If the asymptomatic person is seronegative, then the couple should be counseled regarding preventive measures (condom use) to reduce the chance of transmission.

4. Screening can be selectively offered to those patients as part of a comprehensive evaluation of individuals with a STI and those who are at risk for STIs.
5. Pregnancy applications. The CDC recommends against universal screening in pregnancy. However, screening should be offered to asymptomatic pregnant women whose partners have genital herpes, as well as prenatal patients who are HIV-infected. Discordant couples with an infected man should be counseled regarding the risk of acquiring and transmitting herpes and advised about preventive measures (e.g., abstinence during the third trimester) to avoid an initial primary infection. If the woman is seropositive, she should be counseled regarding the signs and symptoms of genital herpes near term and counseling on plans for route of delivery (see "Pregnancy-Related Issues").
6. Other authors have suggested a broader utilization of serological testing in clinically apparent initial infections, although these applications have not been endorsed or found to be cost effective. These authors have suggested that an HSV-2 titer could be used to counsel women on the likelihood of recurrence (HSV-2 is more likely to occur than HSV-1 infection). Others have recommended routine serological testing for both HSV-1 and HSV-2 antibodies to establish if the clinical outbreak is a primary, non-primary, or a recurrent lesion. The rationale is that if the patient has an HSV infection and if the serology is HSV-1- and HSV-2-negative, then the patient has an initial primary outbreak with exposure during the 14 days before the onset of symptoms. On the other hand, if the serology is HSV-1-positive but HSV-2-negative, then this is an initial non-primary outbreak; in such settings, one could probably come to that conclusion because 80 % of genital herpes is HSV-2. However, the patient would require a repeat testing for HSV-2 in 3 months to confirm this diagnostic impression. If the serology is HSV-2-positive, then the patient has an initial non-primary clinical outbreak of recurrent genital herpes with exposure sometime more 14 days prior.

Diagnosis

The clinical diagnosis of genital herpes can be difficult. This is because the infection presents with "nonclassical" or atypical characteristics or with no symptoms at all. Although the most common cause of genital ulceration is an HSV infection, other etiologies should be considered, including chancroid, traumatic ulceration, primary syphilis, Behçet's syndrome, recurrent aphthous ulcers, fixed drug reaction, Crohn's disease, contact dermatitis, Reiter's syndrome, psoriasis, erythema multiforme, and lichen planus [22]. The clinical diagnosis of genital herpes should always have laboratory confirmation, if possible.

For the last 20 years, the gold standard for diagnosis has been a positive viral culture. However PCR testing is more sensitive than viral culture (see "Testing Techniques"). Viral culture results can be available in 48–72 h and have a false-negative rate of 5–30 %. Patients who present with new onset of genital herpes should also be tested for HIV infection. Testing for other STDs depends on the clinical presentation. Cultures are more likely to detect the virus if they are obtained from the freshly exposed base of a newly ruptured vesicle than if they come from an ulcerated or crusted lesion. Primary infections are more likely to produce positive result than are recurrent infections. Because of the transient nature of viral shedding, a negative culture does not exclude genital herpes. In the patient who has recurrent infections in which isolation of the virus has been difficult, one option is to have the patient return for viral cultures 1 or 2 days into the next outbreak. Another option is to order serological testing for type-specific HSV antibodies to rule out recurrent infections as described earlier.

Treatment

The CDC recommended therapies for initial infections and episodic and suppressive therapies for recurrent infection are displayed in Table 2.3.

Treatment Recommendation for Initial Herpes Genitalis

All patients with initial clinical episodes of symptomatic genital herpes should be treated with an antiviral agent for 7–10 days or until the lesions clear. Local measures, such as saline irrigation, sitz baths, topical anesthesia, use of electric blow dryer on cool setting, and warm compresses are helpful to prevent secondary infection of the lesions and to offer comfort. Careful attention must be paid to limit the spread of infection by autoinoculation. Because the effectiveness of antiviral therapy is dependent on initiation of therapy as early in the clinical stage of disease as possible, treatment with antivirals should be started based on presumptive clinical diagnosis alone, before culture results are available.

The CDC lists three different drugs in four different treatment options for initial clinical episodes of genital herpes (see Table 2.3) [31]. Acyclovir (Zovirax™) was the first drug approved for the treatment of genital herpes. Acyclovir is a purine nucleoside analog that is a competitive inhibitor of viral DNA polymerase. Acyclovir completely inactivates the viral DNA polymerase and terminates viral DNA chain elongation. If given early in the initial stage of HSV infection, acyclovir will reduce the duration of symptoms by an average of 2 days, the time to heal the ulcers by 4 days, and viral shedding by 7 days compared to placebo [4]. In contrast to valacyclovir and famciclovir, acyclovir has poor oral bioavailability and a relatively short

Table 2.3 Treatment of genital herpes—CDC STD treatment guidelines 2010

Agent	Regimen
First clinical episode	
Acyclovir	400 mg orally 3 times a day for 7–10 days[a]
	200 mg orally 5 times a day for 7–10 days[a]
Famciclovir	250 mg orally 3 times a day for 7–10 days[a]
Valacyclovir	1 g orally twice a day for 7–10 days
Severe disease	
Acyclovir	5–10 mg/kg body weight intravenously every 8 h for 2–7 days or until clinical resolution is attained, followed by oral antiviral therapy to complete at least 10 days of therapy
Episodic therapy for recurrent genital herpes	
Acyclovir	400 mg orally 3 times a day for 5 days
	800 mg orally twice a day for 5 days
	800 mg orally three a day for 2 days
Famciclovir	125 mg orally twice a day for 5 days
	1000 mg orally twice daily for 1 day
	500 mg once, followed by 250 mg twice daily for 2 days
Valacyclovir	500 mg orally twice a day for 3 days
	1 g orally once a day for 5 days
Daily suppressive therapy for recurrent genital herpes	
Acyclovir	400 mg orally twice a day
Famciclovir	250 mg orally twice a day
Valacyclovir	500 mg orally once a day
	1 g orally once a day

From Workowski KA, Berman S. Sexually transmitted diseases treatment guidelines, 2010. Centers for Disease Control and Prevention. Division of STD Prevention National Center for HIV/ AIDS, Viral Hepatitis, STD, and TB Prevention. MMWR Recomm Rep 2010;59 (RR-12):1–110
[a]Treatment may be extended, if healing is incomplete after 10 days of therapy

intracellular half-life, which means that acyclovir requires a three-times-a-day oral dosing schedule. For severe herpes infection requiring hospitalization, an intravenous formulation of acyclovir is available. The advantage of oral acyclovir therapy over other oral agents is lower cost, small tablets, and the availability of a liquid formulation. The disadvantages of oral acyclovir are the three-times-a-day dosing frequency.

Valacyclovir (Valtrex™) is a prodrug of acyclovir that is converted to acyclovir in the liver. The oral bioavailability of valacyclovir is much better than acyclovir and approaches the level of intravenous acyclovir. The advantage of valacyclovir is a twice-daily dosing schedule. The disadvantage of valacyclovir is higher cost and unavailability of nonoral formulations.

Famciclovir (Famvir™) is the oral form of penciclovir, a nucleoside analog with properties similar to acyclovir with an improved oral bioavailability [32]. Famciclovir is more expensive than acyclovir.

All oral antiviral agents have been shown to be equally effective [3]. Acyclovir, valacyclovir, and famciclovir have excellent safety profiles with few adverse side effects. It is estimated that more than 80 million people have taken either acyclovir or valacyclovir without significant complications [33]. HSV infections that are resistant to any of the recommended antiviral therapies are rare and generally restricted to immunocompromised patients. If resistance to acyclovir/valacyclovir/famciclovir develops, foscarnet 40 mg/kg body weight intravenously every 8 h is frequently effective. Compounded topical cidofovir gel 1 % applied to lesions once daily for 5 days also might be effective. Acyclovir has been used daily by patients for more than 10 years without any significant adverse effects.

After initiation of therapy, a follow-up visit with the patient should be scheduled in 7–10 days. Test results are usually available by that time, which will provide the caregiver the opportunity to provide more extensive counseling. If examination reveals new lesions or a failure of lesions to reach the crusting phase, then an additional course of antiviral agents should be prescribed.

The use of topical 5 % acyclovir ointment is no longer an FDA-approved as treatment during the initial outbreak because the oral medication is more effective and the use of ointment increases the risk of autoinoculation. Other treatments that should be discouraged owing to documented lack of treatment efficacy include L-lysine, goldenseal, and garlic. Lithium has been noted to decrease frequency of recurrent herpes but has not been proven effective in the treatment of the initial infection [34]. According to the CDC complicated HSV such as aseptic meningitis, disseminated infections, hepatitis, or pneumonitis should be treated initially with acyclovir 5–10 mg/kg IV every 8 h for 2–7 days or until clinical improvement is observed, followed by oral acyclovir to complete at least 10 days of total therapy [35].

Treatment of Recurrent Genital Herpes

If started at the first prodromal symptoms or sign of a recurrence, antiviral treatment of episodic outbreaks will not only reduce the severity and duration of lesions, but may also completely abort the clinical attack, stopping the lesions from progressing beyond the papule stage. The episodic dosing schedules recommended by the CDC for acyclovir (Zovirax) vary by dose and duration of treatment. The episodic recommended dose for valacyclovir and famciclovir are also specified in the CDC recommendation.

The antiviral dosage schedule for suppressive therapy may be different for patients with more frequent (>10) outbreaks annually. All three antivirals appear to be equally effective in preventing outbreaks of genital herpes and reduce asymptomatic viral shedding by 80–90 %.

In serodiscordant couples, suppressive daily antiviral therapy should be strongly considered to reduce further transmission of the infection during the first year when the incidence of asymptomatic viral shedding is highest. However, it should be noted that many couples who are discordant for genital herpes by patient history are found to be concordant by serological testing. Year-long suppressive therapy or longer should be offered to patients with frequent recurrent outbreaks, initial primary infections or patients with stressful or painful recurrences.

Immunocompromised patients are more likely to have prolonged or severe episodes of herpetic outbreak. Higher dose therapy is recommended for episodic therapy for HIV-infected persons, e.g., acyclovir 400 mg orally 3 times daily for 5–10 days; famciclovir 500 mg orally twice daily for 5–10 days; or valacyclovir 1.0 g orally twice a day for 5–10 days. For daily suppressive therapies, acyclovir 400–800 mg is recommended orally twice to 3 times a day or 500-mg doses of famciclovir or valacyclovir orally twice a day.

Counseling

The patient diagnosed with genital herpes may have more difficulty dealing with the psychological impact of the infection than with the physical discomfort. Studies have documented that patients frequently report anger, guilt, decreased self-esteem, loss of interest in intimacy or sex, fear of transmission to their sexual partner, and difficulty with personal relationships because of their diagnosis [36]. Mental and physical health scores in patients diagnosed with genital herpes were lower than the general population [24]. Although it is not currently possible, patients want reassurance that their genital herpes will never recur. Most patients will eventually accept their diagnosis and learn to cope with this chronic condition.

The goals of counseling are patient education, partner notification (in order to break the chain of transmission), education on recognizing outbreak episodes, availability of treatment for viral transmission, as well as risk-reduction maneuvers. The 2006 CDC Guidelines also provide guidance about patient counseling (see Table 2.4). In general, counseling of patients with recurrent herpes should emphasize that there is no known therapy to prevent establishment of latency of the herpes virus in the sensory ganglia of the sacral plexus or to prevent recurrent disease. In other words, there is no cure for herpes. The patient with recurrent disease should avoid intercourse during outbreaks beginning at the onset of prodromal symptoms until crusting over of the lesions several days later. Another option is to use latex condoms at all times, but particularly during genital outbreaks. Information about local self-help and support groups can be helpful.

The major concern of patients with genital herpes remains the fear of transmission to their sexual partners. In serodiscordant couples the transmission is most likely to occur in the first 3–6 months. It is estimated to occur at a rate less than 10 % per year thereafter owing to decreased incidence of viral shedding and clinical outbreaks [19].

Patients should also be advised about the risks of neonatal herpes and the strategies that should be taken to prevent vertical transmission.

Table 2.4 2006 CDC counseling guidelines for patients with herpes genitalis

Information about the natural history of the disease, with emphasis on the potential for
  recurrent episodes, asymptomatic viral shedding, and attendant risks of sexual transmission
Information about episodic or suppressive treatment with antiviral medication to shorten the
  duration of or prevent symptoms
All patients with genital HSV infection should be encouraged to inform their current sex partners
  that they have genital herpes and to inform future partners before initiating a sexual relationship
Persons with genital herpes should be informed that sexual transmission of HSV can occur
  during asymptomatic periods. Asymptomatic viral shedding is more frequent in genital
  IISV-2 infection than in genital HSV-1 infection and is most common in the first 12 months
  following acquisition of HSV-2, but may persist for years, less frequently, in some individuals
Patients should be advised to abstain from sexual activity when lesions or prodromal are present
The risk of HSV sexual transmission can be decreased by the daily use of antiviral agents by the
  infected person
Latex condoms, when used consistently and correctly, can reduce the risk of genital herpes when
  the infected areas are covered or protected by the condom
Sex partners of infected persons should be advised that they might themselves be infected even if
  they have no symptoms. Type-specific serological testing of asymptomatic partners of
  persons with genital herpes can determine whether risk for HSV acquisition exists
The risk of neonatal infection should be explained to all patients, including men. Pregnant
  women and women of childbearing age who have genital herpes should inform their
  providers who care for them during pregnancy, as well as those who will care for their
  newborns infants. Pregnant women who are not infected with HSV-2 should be advised to
  avoid intercourse during the third trimester with men who have genital herpes. Similarly,
  pregnant women who are not infected with HSV-1 should be counseled to avoid genital
  exposure to HSV-1 (e.g., oral sex with a partner with oral herpes and vaginal intercourse with
  a partner with genital HSV-1 infection) during the third trimester
Asymptomatic persons diagnosed with HSV-2 infection by type-specific serological testing
  should receive the same counseling messages as persons with symptomatic infection. In
  addition, such persons should be taught about the clinical manifestations of genital herpes

HSV herpes simplex virus, *HIV* human immunodeficiency virus

Pregnancy-Related Issues

About 22 % of pregnant women are infected with HSV-2 and 2 % will acquire HSV during pregnancy [37]. Initial HSV infection is particularly severe if it develops during pregnancy; pregnancy does not appear to increase the rate of recurrence of maternal outbreaks.

The most serious consequences of maternal infection are adverse fetal impacts and newborn infection. An initial maternal genital herpes outbreak in the first trimester of pregnancy has been associated with fetal chorioretinitis, microcephaly, and skin lesions but not spontaneous abortion or fetal death [38]. Neonatal HSV infection occurs in about 1,500 cases each year [39, 40]. Neonatal HSV infection has three clinical presentations: disseminated disease involving multiple organs, such as the liver, lungs, and the central nervous system (25 % of cases); disease localized to the skin, eyes, and mouth (40 % of cases); and localized central nervous system disease (35 % of cases). Up to 30 % of infected neonates will die and up to 40 % of survivors will have neurological damage, despite antiviral therapy [40].

Infection can be transmitted from the mother to her fetus/newborn in three ways: transplacentally (5–8 %), intrapartum exposure (85 %), or postpartum exposure (8–10 %) [39]. The likelihood and severity of neonatal infection is influenced by the mother's antibody status. If a woman develops initial primary infection during pregnancy, there is a 5 % chance of transplacental transmission to the baby.

Most neonatal infections result from fetal exposure during delivery. The remaining confirmed cases of neonatal herpes may have been acquired postnatally, either from the mother, a relative, or hospital worker as a result of oral contact or contact with an infected finger (whitlow) [41].

Neonatal herpes infections develop in 30–50 % of exposed infants whose mothers have an initial primary infection near time of delivery [10]. The risk of neonatal herpes from an asymptomatic mother with a history of recurrent HSV at term or who acquire HSV in the first-half of pregnancy is much lower (<1 %). Only infants delivered to women who are actively shedding from recurrent infections at the time of delivery will acquire infection. It has been estimated by PCR techniques that 6–10 % of HSV-2-seropositive women shed virus in labor [42]. However, because of the ubiquitous nature of this infection, more neonatal infections result from recurrent infections than from initial maternal infections. Infrequently, the infant may be infected by a caregiver with oral herpetic lesion or herpes whitlow, which involves the distal fingers.

The role of testing for HSV infection in pregnancy is under debate. The cost-effectiveness of routine HSV screening in pregnancy is controversial [43, 44].

It has been suggested that type-specific HSV-2 serology testing be performed on women who have no personal history of HSV but whose partners are known to be infected. Women who tested negative could be advised to avoid sexual contact, at least during the third trimester and encouraged to use condoms (or abstinence) throughout the rest of pregnancy. The effectiveness of antiviral therapy for the partner to decrease the risk of HSV transmission to pregnant women has not been studied.

Women who develop primary HSV infection during pregnancy should be treated with acyclovir [40, 45]. Acyclovir, valacyclovir, and famciclovir are classified as pregnancy category B drugs by the FDA. More than 1200 pregnancy outcomes have been followed in infants exposed in utero at all stages of fetal development to acyclovir. No significant differences in rates of birth defects or adverse pregnancy outcomes have been reported [33]. Experience with valacyclovir and famciclovir is too limited in the CDC estimation to provide information about the safety of its use in pregnancy.

For women who are known to have recurrent outbreaks of genital lesions, suppressive therapy with antiviral agents starting at 36 weeks gestational age has also been shown to reduce the rate of symptomatic outbreaks and asymptomatic shedding and the need for cesarean section [46]. Therefore the American College of Obstetricians and Gynecologists advise beginning acyclovir 400 mg three-time-a-day or valacylovir 500 mg twice a day from 36 weeks until delivery [47]. The use of scalp monitors in labor should be discouraged in women who are known to shed HSV, but the American College of Obstetricians and Gynecologists says the use is not contraindicated if needed to assess fetal condition adequately in women with a history of HSV but without symptoms or lesions.

Cesarean delivery is recommended for women who have active genital lesions or prodromal symptoms at the time of rupture of membranes or labor. Operative delivery has been shown to reduce the risk of transmission significantly in initial infection. Vaginal delivery is recommended for women who do not have lesions or symptoms at the time of delivery. C-section is not needed if the patient has lesions in extra-genital areas, such as the buttocks or legs. The lesions can be covered and the patients can be allowed to deliver vaginally.

The pediatrician should always be informed of the maternal/patient history of herpes and the status of the mother at the time of delivery. Acyclovir may be recommended if the mother acquired the infection during pregnancy (especially third trimester) pending the results of the maternal and/or newborn culture.

Breastfeeding is not contraindicated except in mothers who have active HSV infections on the nipple or other sites on their breasts. Mothers should use caution when handling newborns and may take antiviral therapies when breastfeeding to diminish shedding.

Partner Notification and Reporting Requirements

HSV is not a reportable disease in most states. Patients should be advised to talk with their sex partners about their diagnosis. If the partner is infected with the same HSV type, no precautions need to be taken. Patients should understand most infected partners are not aware that they carry the virus. All new sex partners should be informed of the potential for infection and that safer sex practices may reduce, but do not eliminate, the possibility of transmission.

Prevention

Latex condoms are impermeable to passage of the 160 nm HSV-2. In 2002, a National Institutes of Health expert panel reviewed the literature and found that there was not sufficient data to allow it to form any conclusions about the effectiveness/ineffectiveness of correct and consistent condom usage in reducing the risk of genital herpes infection [6]. However, a subsequent study of discordant couples found that when condoms were used more than 25 % of the time, the risk of transmission to an uninfected woman was reduced by more than 90 % (see Chap. 14) [12]. More recently, analysis of data collected as part of a clinical trial of an ineffective candidate vaccine for HSV-2 revealed that those who reported more frequent condom use were at lower risk for acquiring HSV-2 than those who used condoms less frequently [48]. Counseling for consistent condom use is needed because, despite the fact that there is a risk of transmission from asymptomatic shedding, couples are less likely to use condoms when active lesions are absent [49].

Chronic suppressive therapy is effective in preventing both clinical recurrences and asymptomatic viral shedding. Avoiding sexual contact during episodes of known clinical outbreaks will prevent transmission of HSV. Several vaccines are currently being tested in Phase III clinical trials but the development of an effective vaccine to prevent genital HSV has been challenging (see Chap. 15) [50].

Selected Resources

American Social Health Association

A comprehensive resource for patients, their partners, and care givers. Offers herpes prevention, screening, and disease management information.
Home of the National Herpes Resource Center
Web site: http://www.ashastd.org/std-sti/Herpes.html
Phone: 800-783-9877 for a free catalog

The International Herpes Management Forum

Wide range of herpes issues for both physicians and patients.
Web site: http://www.ihmf.org/Patient/PatientResources.asp

Fact Sheet on Genital Herpes

From the CDC National Center for HIV, STD, and TB Prevention in the Division of Sexually Transmitted Diseases.
Web site: http://www.cdc.gov/std/Herpes/STDFact-Herpes.htm

National STD Hotline

Health information hotline dedicated to providing accurate, basic information, referrals, and educational materials on a wide variety of STDs. Hotline specialists answer basic questions about STDs and refer callers to public health clinics and other local resources.
Phone: 800-232-4636 (24 h in English and Spanish).

National Herpes Hotline

Operated by American Social Health Association (ASHA) as part of the National Herpes Resource Center.
Free counseling on herpes as well as referrals.
A list of local support groups is available at: http://www.ashastd.org/hrc/help grp1. html
Phone: 919-361-8488
(9 AM–6 PM Eastern Standard Time, Monday through Friday) Web site: http:// www.herpesonline.org

References

1. Roizman B, Whitley RJ. The nine ages of herpes simplex virus. Herpes. 2001;8:23–7.
2. Xu F, Sternberg MR, Kottiri BJ, et al. Trends in herpes simplex virus type 1 and type 2 seroprevalence in the United States. JAMA. 2006;296(8):964–73.
3. Yeung-Yue KA, Brentjens MH, Lee PC, Tyring SK. Herpes simplex viruses 1 and 2. Dermatol Clin. 2002;20:249–66.
4. Mertz GJ, Benedetti J, Ashley R, Selke SA, Corey L. Risk factors for the sexual transmission of genital herpes. Ann Intern Med. 1992;116:197–202.
5. Corey L, Wald A, Patel R, et al. Once-daily valacyclovir to reduce the risk of transmission of genital herpes. N Engl J Med. 2004;350:11–20.
6. National Institute of Allergy and Infectious Diseases. Workshop summary: scientific evidence on condom effectiveness for sexually transmitted disease (STD) prevention. Washington, DC: National Institutes of Health, Department of Health Services; 2001. Available from: http://www.niaid.nih.gov/dmid/stds/condomreport.pdf. Accessed 4 June 2005.
7. World Health Organization. Global prevalence and incidence of selected curable sexually transmitted infections: overview and estimates. Geneva: World Health Organization; 2001. Available from: http://www.who.int/emc-documents/STIs/whocdscsredc200110c.html. Accessed 10 July 2005.
8. Schacker T. The role of HSV in the transmission and progression of HIV. Herpes. 2001;8:46–9.
9. Schacker T, Ryncarz AJ, Goddard J, Diem K, Shaughnessy M, Corey L. Frequent recovery of HIV-1 from genital herpes simplex virus lesions in HIV-1-infected men. JAMA. 1998;280:61–6.
10. Mole L, Ripich S, Margolis D, Holodniy M. The impact of active herpes simplex virus infection on human immunodeficiency virus load. J Infect Dis. 1997;176:766–70.
11. Wald A, Link K. Risk of human immunodeficiency virus infection in herpes simplex virus type 2-seropositive persons: a meta-analysis. J Infect Dis. 2002;185:45–52.
12. Wald A. Herpes simplex virus type 2 transmission: risk factors and virus shedding. Herpes. 2004;11:130A–7.
13. Wald A, Langenberg AG, Link K, et al. Effect of condoms on reducing the transmission of herpes simplex virus type 2 from men to women. JAMA. 2001;285:3100–6.
14. Cherpes TL, Meyn LA, Krohn MA, Hillier SL. Risk factors for infection with herpes simplex virus type 2: role of smoking, douching, uncircumcised males, and vaginal flora. Sex Transm Dis. 2003;30:405–10.
15. Langenberg AG, Corey L, Ashley RL, Leong WP, Straus SE. A prospective study of new infections with herpes simplex virus type 1 and type 2. Chiron HSV Vaccine Study Group. N Engl J Med. 1999;341:1432–8.
16. Lafferty WE, Downey L, Celum C, Wald A. Herpes simplex virus type 1 as a cause of genital herpes: impact on surveillance and prevention. J Infect Dis. 2000;181:1454–7.
17. Wald A, Zeh J, Selke S, et al. Reactivation of genital herpes simplex virus type 2 infection in asymptomatic seropositive persons. N Engl J Med. 2000;342:844–50.
18. Wald A, Corey L, Cone R, Hobson A, Davis G, Zeh J. Frequent genital herpes simplex virus 2 shedding in immunocompetent women. Effect of acyclovir treatment. J Clin Invest. 1997;99:1092–7.
19. Bryson Y, Dillon M, Bernstein DI, Radolf J, Zakowski P, Garratty E. Risk of acquisition of genital herpes simplex virus type 2 in sex partners of persons with genital herpes: a prospective couple study. J Infect Dis. 1993;167:942–6.
20. Koelle DM, Benedetti J, Langenberg A, Corey L. Asymptomatic reactivation of herpes simplex virus in women after the first episode of genital herpes. Ann Intern Med. 1992;116:433–7.
21. Benedetti J, Corey L, Ashley R. Recurrence rates in genital herpes after symptomatic first episode infection. Ann Intern Med. 1994;121:847–54.

22. Kimberlin DW, Rouse DJ. Clinical practice. Genital herpes. N Engl J Med. 2004;350:1970–7.
23. Corey L, Adams HG, Brown ZA, Holmes KK. Genital herpes simplex virus infections: clinical manifestations, course, and complications. Ann Intern Med. 1983;98:958–72.
24. Patel R, Boselli F, Cairo I, Barnett G, Price M, Wulf HC. Patients' perspectives on the burden of recurrent genital herpes. Int J STD AIDS. 2001;12:640–5.
25. Sweet RL, Gibbs RS. Herpes simplex virus infection. In: Sweet RL, Gibbs RS, editors. Infectious diseases of the female genital tract. 4th ed. Philadelphia, PA: Lippincott, Williams & Wilkins; 2002. p. 101–17.
26. Kessler HA, Baker DA, Brown ZA, Leone PA. Herpesvirus management: special considerations for the female patient. A monograph based on a symposium held May 6, New York, NY: New World Health; 2002.
27. Ebel C, Wald A. Managing herpes: how to live and love with a chronic STD. 3rd ed. Research Park Triangle, NC: American Social Health Association; 2002.
28. Kaufman RH, Gardner HL, Rawls WE, Dixon RE, Young RL. Clinical features of herpes genitalis. Cancer Res. 1973;33:1446–51.
29. Benedetti JK, Zeh J, Corey L. Clinical reactivation of genital herpes simplex virus infection decreases in frequency over time. Ann Intern Med. 1999;131:14–20.
30. Ashley-Morrow R, Krantz E, Wald A. Time course of seroconversion by HerpesSelect ELISA after acquisition of genital herpes simplex virus type 1 (HSV-1) or HSV-2. Sex Transm Dis. 2003;30:310.
31. Centers for Disease Control and Prevention. Sexually transmitted diseases treatment guidelines 2002. MMWR Recomm Rep. 2002;51:1–78.
32. Diaz-Mitoma F, Sibbald RG, Shafran SD, Boon R, Saltzman RL. Oral famciclovir for the suppression of recurrent genital herpes: a randomized controlled trial. Collaborative Famciclovir Genital Herpes Research Group. JAMA. 1998;280:887–92.
33. Tyring SK, Baker D, Snowden W. Valacyclovir for herpes simplex virus infection: longterm safety and sustained efficacy after 20 years experience with acyclovir. J Infect Dis. 2002;186:S40–6.
34. Parks DG, Greenway FL, Pack AT. Prevention of recurrent herpes simplex type II infection with lithium carbonate. Med Sci Res. 1988;16:971–2.
35. Workowski KA, Berman S. Sexually transmitted disease treatment guidelines. 2010. Centers for Disease Control and Prevention. Division of STD Prevention National Center for HIV/AIDS, Viral Hepatitis, STD and TB Prevention. MMWR Recomm Rep. 2010;59(RR-12):1–110.
36. Alexander L, Naisbett B. Patient and physician partnerships in managing genital herpes. J Infect Dis. 2002;186:S57–65.
37. Brown ZA, Gardella C, Wald A, Morrow RA, Corey L. Genital herpes complicating pregnancy. Obstet Gynecol. 2005;106(4):845–56.
38. Eskild A, Jeansson S, Stray-Pedersen B, Jenum PA. Herpes simplex virus type-2 infection in pregnancy: no risk of fetal death: results from a nested case–control study within 35,940 women. BJOG. 2002;109:1030–5.
39. Brown Z. Preventing herpes simplex virus transmission to the neonate. Herpes. 2004;11:175A–86.
40. Kimberlin DW. Neonatal herpes simplex infection. Clin Microbiol Rev. 2004;17(1):1–13.
41. Smith JR, Cowan FM, Munday P. The management of herpes simplex virus infection in pregnancy. Br J Obstet Gynaecol. 1998;105:255–60.
42. Watts DH, Brown ZA, Money D, et al. A double-blind, randomized, placebo-controlled trial of acyclovir in late pregnancy for the reduction of herpes simplex virus shedding and cesarean delivery. Am J Obstet Gynecol. 2003;188:836–43.
43. Thung SF, Grobman WA. The cost-effectiveness of routine antenatal screening for maternal herpes simplex virus-1 and -2 antibodies. Am J Obstet Gynecol. 2005;192:483–8.
44. Baker D, Brown Z, Hollier LM, et al. Cost-effectiveness of herpes simplex virus type 2 serologic testing and antiviral therapy in pregnancy. Am J Obstet Gynecol. 2004;191:2074–84.

45. American College of Obstetricians and Gynecologists. ACOG Practice Bulletin. Management of herpes in pregnancy. Number 8 October 1999. Clinical management guidelines for obstetrician-gynecologists. Int J Gynaecol Obstet. 2000;68:165–73.
46. Sheffield JS, Hollier LM, Hill JB, Stuart GS, Wendel GD. Acyclovir prophylaxis to prevent herpes simplex virus recurrence at delivery: a systematic review. Obstet Gynecol. 2003;102:1396–403.
47. American College of Obstetricians and Gynecologists (ACOG). Management of herpes in pregnancy. Washington, DC: ACOG; 2007 (ACOG practice bulletin; no. 82).
48. Wald A, Langenberg AG, Krantz E, et al. The relationship between condom use and herpes simplex virus acquisition. Ann Intern Med. 2005;143(10):707–13.
49. Rana RK, Pimenta JM, Rosenberg DM, et al. Sexual behaviour and condom use among individuals with a history of symptomatic genital herpes. Sex Transm Infect. 2006;82(1):69–74.
50. National Institute of Allergy and Infectious Disease. Genital herpes. Washington DC: National Institutes of Health, Department of Health Services; 2011. Available from: http://www.niaid.nih.gov/topics/genitalherpes/research/researchreport.pdf. Accessed 24 May 2012.

Chapter 3
Chlamydia

Albert John Phillips

Introduction

Chlamydia trachomatis is the most commonly reported infectious disease in the United States and is the most common sexually transmitted bacterial infection [1]. A large reservoir of infection sustains the continued spread of *C. trachomatis* because chlamydial infections rarely cause symptoms in women, they have a long incubation period, and the infection persists for at least several months. The annual cost of chlamydial infections and their sequellae in the United States is estimated to be 647 million dollars (in year 2008 dollars) [2, 3].

Fast Facts

- Chlamydia is the most commonly reported bacterial infection, with an estimated three million new cases each year.
- Adolescents and young adults are most commonly infected with *C. trachomatis*.
- By age 30, 50 % of US women carry antibodies indicating prior exposure.
- The majority of infections with *C. trachomatis* in both men and women are asymptomatic.
- Up to 40 % of untreated chlamydial cervicitis cases will ascend into the upper genital tract, where considerable tubal damage can occur with very few symptoms.

A.J. Phillips, MD (✉)
Obstetrics & Gynecology, Keck School of Medicine, University of Southern California,
1301 20th Street, Suite 270, Santa Monica, CA 90404, USA
e-mail: albertjphillips@gmail.com

N.S. Skolnik et al. (eds.), *Sexually Transmitted Diseases: A Practical Guide for Primary Care*, Current Clinical Practice, DOI 10.1007/978-1-62703-499-9_3,
© Springer Science+Business Media New York 2013

- All sexually active women under age 26 should be screened at least annually. Such screening has been demonstrated to reduce the incidence of upper tract infection.
- All pregnant women should be routinely tested at the first prenatal visit. Pregnant women aged 25 years and younger and those at increased risk should be retested during the third trimester to prevent maternal postnatal complications and chlamydial infection in the infant [4].

Prevalence/Incidence

In 2000, the Centers for Disease Control and Prevention (CDC) required states to report all cases of chlamydia. Even with this requirement in place, it is believed that chlamydial infections are significantly underreported because of sporadic screening. In 2010, an estimated 1.31 million cases were reported to the CDC, up from 1.24 million in 2009 [1]. Local studies demonstrated that the prevalence of infected and untreated cases equaled or exceeded the number of cases that were diagnosed and treated [5]. Nearly 75 % of cases occur in the 15–24-year-old age group [6]. The World Health Organization (WHO) estimated that 98 million new infections with C. trachomatis occurred worldwide in 2005 [7].

Women primarily are most likely to be diagnosed with infection and to suffer more severe, long-term consequences. Chlamydial infection rates were nearly 3 times higher in women than in men in 2010 in the United States [1]. The prevalence of active infection in sexually active, asymptomatic, nonpregnant women in the general population is between 3 and 5 % [8]. The National Longitudinal Study of Adolescent Health tested the urine of over 12,000 young adults age 18–26 and found the overall prevalence of chlamydial infection was 4.19 %, and ranged from 1.94 to 12.54 % depending on demographics [9]. Women in family planning clinics have a background rate of 2.8–9.4 %, while patients in STD clinics are found to have a 15–33 % incidence [8].

In the general population, men have the same prevalence of chlamydial infections as women (3–5 %). In STD clinics, the prevalence rates among men are 15–20 %, which is slightly less than the rates among women [8]. Chlamydial infections are found in 13–15 % of sexually active men in adolescent clinics. The prevalence of chlamydial infection in men who have sex with men (MSM) varies by anatomical site: rectal 7.9 %, urethral 5.2 %, and pharyngeal 1.4 % [10]. In asymptomatic MSM who were screened, 11 % were found to have to be positive for either chlamydia or gonorrhea [11]. Even though the majority of chlamydial infections are found in younger women, increases of infections have been seen in MSM. In this group, more than 50 % of chlamydial infections are in the rectum or pharynx [10].

Chlamydia is often found as a co-infection with gonorrhea in both men and women. Between 30 and 50 % of patients who have gonococcal infections also have infection with C. trachomatis. However, because the background incidence of gonorrhea is so much lower (<0.5 %), it is far less likely that a person infected with *C. trachomatis* will also have gonococcal infections. There also appears to be a difference in the rate of co-infection between sexes. A recent study showed a 5.4 % co-infection rate in males younger than 26, while females under 26 had a rate of 2 % [12].

Risk Factors

Specific historical and behavioral factors place a patient at an increased risk for acquisition of *C. trachomatis*. The classic risk factors for chlamydial infection include age less than 26, low socioeconomic status, minority group member, multiple sexual partners, and new partners. Age is an important risk factor because *C. trachomatis* typically infects the columnar cells of the cervix. In younger women, columnar cells are more likely to be on the ectocervix (ectopy), where they can be exposed to semen carrying the organism. As a women age, the columnar cells are located higher in the cervical canal. Combination hormonal contraceptive use apparently increases cervical ectopy and has been a proposed risk factor chlamydial infection [13].

African-American women are disproportionately impacted by chlamydia. In 2010, the rate of chlamydia infection among black women was 8 times higher than in white women [1].

Infectivity and Transmission

C. trachomatis is a relatively infectious agent. Over two-thirds of female partners of men with culture-positive chlamydial urethritis have chlamydial infection themselves [8]. The single exposure male-to-female transmission rate has been estimated to be 40 %, and the female-to-male transmission rate has been estimated to be 32 % [8]. Other investigators have found that transmission rates between sexes are equivalent [14]. Vertical transmission of *C. trachomatis* is more efficient than horizontal transmission. Over 60 % of newborns who deliver through a chlamydia-infected cervix will acquire the infection [8].

Etiology

C. trachomatis is one of four species of the genus Chlamydia. It is responsible for a wide range of infections including trachoma (a chronic conjunctivitis, which is the leading preventable cause of blindness worldwide), newborn conjunctivitis, and genital infections in women and men. *C. trachomatis* is an obligate intracellular organism, dependent on the host cell's adenosine triphosphate (ATP) production. *C. trachomatis* has a unique life cycle, which differentiates it from all other microorganisms. Infection begins when elemental bodies (EBs) attach to specific receptors found on nonciliated columnar or cuboidal epithelium of the host. This type of epithelium is located in the endocervix, endometrium, fallopian tube and urethra, making those sites vulnerable to infection.

The host cell ingests the organism by a chlamydia-specific phagocytic process. After phagocytosis, the EB exists within a cytoplasmic vacuole or phagosome, where it is protected from host defense systems. Within the phagosome, the EB transforms into a reticulate body (RB), which is the form the organism assumes in order to multiply. It multiplies by binary fusion, after duplicating its own DNA, RNA, and proteins by using host ATP. The RBs then reorganize back into EBs, the infectious form of the organism. Ultimately, the host cell undergoes either lysis or exocytosis with release of the EBs, which infects adjacent cells and restarts the cycle. This process takes 2–3 days.

C. trachomatis has features of both bacteria and virus. *C. trachomatis* has a cell wall like gram-negative bacteria but it cannot synthesize its own ATP or grow on artificial media, hence its similarity with a virus. Because of its unique developmental cycle, it is taxonomically classified in a separate order. The chemical composition of the cell wall of the EB is quite similar to that of gram-negative bacteria. The cell wall of the RB contains less phospholipid than the EB. RBs are highly labile and do not survive outside of the host cell. However, the EB is relatively stable in extracellular environments because its envelope is strengthened due to cysteine proteins that are cross-linked by disulfide bonds, providing the EB structural integrity and resistance.

C. trachomatis is currently classified into 15 serotypes (serovars). Typically, different serovars are associated with specific clinical diseases. The different serovars of *C. trachomatis* within groups have not been shown to have different clinical courses [15].

Clinical Manifestations

The range of infections with *C. trachomatis* is impressive (see Table 3.1). The predominant infections are urethritis, cervicitis, and proctitis, but chlamydial infection can spread locally to the Bartholin's glands, endosalpinges, or epididymis. In pregnancy, chlamydial infection is a risk factor for low birth weight infants and preterm delivery. Postpartum, an infected woman is at increased risk for developing endometritis. Her newborn can develop conjunctivitis and pneumonia. Men who have chlamydial urethritis are at risk for developing Reiter's syndrome. Each of these clinical infections has a wide spectrum of initial presenting symptoms, ranging from no symptoms to noticeable discomfort and pain.

Table 3.1 Clinical manifestations of *C. trachomatis* infections

Women	Men	Newborn
Demonstrated		
Cervicitis	Urethritis	Conjunctivitis
Urethritis	Epididymitis	Pneumonia
Acute urethral syndrome	Prostatitis	Otitis media
Proctitis	Proctitis	
Endometritis	Infertility	
Salpingitis	Conjunctivitis	
Perihepatitis	Reiter's syndrome	
Conjunctivitis		
Ectopic pregnancy		
Infertility		
Chronic pelvic pain		
Reiter's syndrome		
Suggested		
Preterm labor		
Preterm delivery		
Premature rupture membranes		
Postpartum endometritis		

Infections in Women

Cervicitis

The cervix is the most common site of infection for women. Women with chlamydial cervicitis generally are asymptomatic or report only nonspecific symptoms, such as vaginal discharge or postcoital spotting or bleeding. Two-thirds of infected women have no signs or symptoms. Furthermore, because the incubation period for *C. trachomatis* is 6–14 days, women may not relate their subtle symptoms to a distant exposure. Secondary or related infections (trichomoniasis or gonorrhea) are generally the etiology for complaints in women with symptoms.

On speculum exam, the chlamydia-infected cervix may appear entirely normal or may have a mucopurulent discharge and eroded friable appearance. *C. trachomatis* infects only columnar cells in the cervical squamocolumnar region or in the endocervix. In women with cervical ectopy and mucopurulent cervicitis, *C. trachomatis* should be considered, but mucopurulent cervicitis should not be used as definitive evidence of chlamydial cervicitis. The presence of leukocytes in endocervical samples studied under magnification is a better predictor of chlamydial infection, when other causes have been ruled out. Testing with sensitive laboratory-based tests (see below) is needed to confirm the diagnosis.

Bimanual exam should always be performed after appropriate specimens have been collected. Gentle exam for cervical motion tenderness should be performed to assess possible upper tract involvement (see Section on "Salpingitis"). Once chlamydial infection is suspected, concrete questions should be asked about sexual practices to identify other sites that might be involved.

Urethritis/Urethral Syndrome

Women with chlamydial urethritis are generally asymptomatic. Those who have acute infections may complain of dysuria, slight discharge in urine, or urinary frequency. A woman with chlamydial urethritis/urethral syndrome will note that her symptoms are focused in the suprapubic area and start after she has finished voiding, which may help distinguish that infection from bacterial cystitis. Conventional urinalysis and culture testing will reveal sterile pyuria. Because only selective antibiotics will treat chlamydial infections, the symptoms will not resolve with typical antibiotic therapies for bacterial cystitis. The differential diagnosis includes infection with Mycoplasma or Ureaplasma as well as urethral trauma and atrophic urethritis. Direct testing for *C. trachomatis* can be done on specimens obtained by urethral swabs or on urine from the first part of the stream. It is rare for chlamydial urethritis to exist independent of a cervical infection in a woman.

Bartholinitis

The Bartholin's gland and ducts are lined with columnar epithelium and are susceptible to infection with *C. trachomatis*. It has been estimated that 30 % of Bartholin's gland infections are abscesses initiated by chlamydial infection, although the absolute contribution is not known [16, 17]. Women with Bartholin's abscesses complain of acute onset of vulvar pain and swelling, which becomes quite intense as the abscess expands. Generally treatment required for abscess is incision and marsupialization and adjuvant antibiotic treatment is not recommended. However, 8 % of patients presenting with Bartholin's abscess had chlamydia found in either the abscess or the uterus [18]. Therefore it would be prudent to test for chlamydia in these situations.

Salpingitis

Ascending infection from the lower genital tract occurs in approximately 10 % of patients with cervicitis. Sperm has been implicated in the transport of *C. trachomatis* into the upper genital tract in women. Symptoms may appear at any time during a woman's menstrual cycle, in contrast to gonococcal pelvic inflammatory disease (PID), which classically develops at the end of a woman's menses. The clinical presentation of chlamydial salpingitis is much more subtle than gonococcal salpingitis, because the fallopian tubes may not be distended with chlamydial infection even though the endosalpinges may suffer profound architectural damage as a result of chlamydial heat shock proteins. Women with significant upper tract infection may be asymptomatic or have only mild flu-like discomforts that they attribute to other causes. Because of this very unremarkable clinical symptomatology and the relative paucity of clinical findings on examination and laboratory testing, the CDC revised its requirements for the criteria of PID to lower the threshold for diagnosis. See Chap. 5 (Upper Genital Infections in Women) for more information about diagnosis and treatment.

Infections in Men

Chlamydial Urethritis

Nongonococcal urethritis is most commonly caused by *C. trachomatis*. The typical incubation period from exposure to infection is 1–2 weeks. Men who are symptomatic generally present with complaints of dysuria, urinary frequency, and urethral discharge. The discharge is greatest in the morning when it can be milked from the urethra. A diagnosis of nongonococcal urethritis is made when a gram-stain of the discharge demonstrates 4 or more white blood cells (WBCs) per field on high power (×1,000) and there are no diplococci or first voided urine has positive leukocyte esterase and microscopic examination reveals 10 or more WBCs per high power field [19, 20]. Unfortunately, urethritis is often asymptomatic; therefore, infected men are a major reservoir for infection of their sexual partners [14].

Prostatitis

The symptoms associated with prostatitis are perineal pain, back pain, and pain with urination or ejaculation. Acute prostatitis in young men can occur with *C. trachomatis*. The role of *C. trachomatis* in chronic prostatitis is not so clear. Over one-quarter of men with nonbacterial chronic prostatitis were found to have chlamydial antigens and 80 % showed cures after treatment with doxycycline [21]. More than one in 5 men with chronic prostatitis with inflammation seen on prostatic secretions had evidence of chlamydial infection [22]. These results suggest that *C. trachomatis* may be one of the causative agents of chronic prostatitis [22].

Epididymitis

Tenderness with swelling in the testicle is a sign of epididymitis. Acute epididymitis more commonly occurs in younger men. Other infectious etiologics for epididymitis include *N. gonorrhea* and *E. coli*. Chlamydial epididymitis has a milder course than other etiologies. Chronic epididymitis is defined as testicular pain persisting for at least 3 months. Because of the indolent nature of chlamydial infections, a patient with chronic epididymitis can also have a scrotal mass. Male infertility may be associated with chlamydial infections because the inflammatory process may damage the epididymis and the sperm collection tubules. Men with fertility problems have been found by serology to have more likely had a previous infection of Chlamydia, but definitive proof is not yet been established [23].

Infections in Men or Women

Proctitis

Chlamydial proctitis can occur in women and MSM who practice receptive anal intercourse. *C. trachomatis* was found in specimens from 5 % of rectums and 13 % of cervixes of 115 consecutive women presenting for examination. Rectal bleeding and microscopic evidence of proctitis without diarrhea was commonly found [24]. With MSM, the infection is due to unprotected anal intercourse. Chlamydial proctitis has been found in 15 % of asymptomatic MSM males [25]. With symptomatic men and women, sigmoidoscopy and appropriate testing for infectious organisms is required. Human immunodeficiency virus (HIV) antibody status should be established. If the patient is HIV-infected, uncommon pathogens need to be considered. With negative HIV tests, treatment for both gonorrhea and chlamydial infections is appropriate.

Reactive Arthritis/Reiter's Syndrome

Reactive arthritis is an inflammatory synovitis in which no viable organisms can be isolated from the joint and is precipitated by an immunologic response to an infectious agent. Reiter's syndrome is composed of a triad of conjunctivitis, urethritis, and arthritis. Often individuals will not manifest all elements of the triad. Men are approximately 9 times more likely to develop Reiter's syndrome than women. Multiple joint involvement is common, usually affecting the knees or feet. Joint symptoms develop 2–4 weeks after urogenital infection, but 10 % of affected individuals have no history of urethritis. Conjunctivitis and associated iritis and uveitis usually develop after the arthritis. A scaly skin rash (keratoderma blennorrhagica) on the palms or soles is also seen.

Many organisms have been implicated in reactive arthritis and Reiter's syndrome, including *C. trachomatis*. In genetically susceptible individuals, the immune system reacts to the infectious agent leading to the inflammatory response in the synovial surface [26]. Evidence of urogenital *C. trachomatis* was found in 36–61 % of cases of Reiter's syndrome and chlamydial inclusions may be found in the fibroblast-like synovial cells [27].

Chlamydial Infection in the Newborn

Neonatal chlamydial infection usually develops from vertical transmission. In one study, 6 out of 10 infants who delivered vaginally to mothers with infections had serologic evidence of infection. The clinical manifestations varied; 18 % of exposed infants developed neonatal conjunctivitis and 16 % had pneumonia. Subclinical rectal and vaginal infections also occurred in the newborn [28]. Although the most common method of transmission is thought to be direct contract as the fetus delivers through an infected cervix, there have been reported instances where neonatal infection occurred with Cesarean section delivery, with and without ruptured membranes [29].

Chlamydial neonatal conjunctivitis has an incubation period of 10–14 days. The orbit of the eye swells and exudates are seen. *C. trachomatis* will be found in a high proportion of specimens. Because *C. trachomatis* can also be found in the nasopharynx, systemic treatment is required rather than a local ophthalmic solution. Twenty percent of untreated neonates will develop neonatal pneumonia without conjunctivitis [30]. Pneumonia occurs between the 4th and 12th week of life, with the majority of newborns becoming symptomatic by the eighth week of life. They may present with failure to thrive, decreased appetite, and some lethargy. More severely infected infants will present with tachypnea and a staccato-like cough. Upper respiratory symptoms include congestion and nasal passage obstruction without significant nasal discharge. Serious acute complications may require prolonged hospitalization and intubation with ventilator support. Diagnosis can be made by assessing *C. trachomatis* IgM antibody titers. Long-term complications of pneumonia can include abnormal pulmonary function tests and asthma [31].

Testing Techniques

There is a wide spectrum of technologies available today to detect *C. trachomatis* infection. These tests can be used on a wide variety of specimens. However, there are considerable differences in their respective abilities to detect infection. Selection of the appropriate test, and the need for possible confirmatory tests, depends in large part upon the prevalence of the infection in local populations. Therefore, familiarity with the different tests and their properties is needed to enhance detection of infected individuals and to reduce false positive results. See Table 3.2 for a summary of the different tests and testing sites by indication.

The most common tests used today are non-culture tests, although tissue culture tests are still required for some applications. Non-culture tests use a variety of techniques that bind tags to specific chlamydia proteins. The most sensitive and accurate of the non-culture tests are the nucleic acid amplification tests (NAATs). NAATs test for a unique nucleic acid (DNA or RNA) of the chlamydial organism or use a probe that is attached to the target nucleic acid. NAATs are very sensitive; they can detect a single gene copy. NAATs are also very specific.

There are several types of NAATs. The two most commonly used tests are the polymerase chain reaction (PCR) and ligase chain reaction (LCR) tests. PCR amplifies the nucleic acids found on the *C. trachomatis* EB. PCR has a sensitivity of 90 % and a specificity of 99–100 %. PCR tests are approved for cervical, male urethral swabs, and male urine specimens. LCR has an overall sensitivity of 94 % and a specificity of 99–100 %. LCR can be used to test urethral and cervical swabs, as well as first voided urine. More recently, LCR has been refined for use with liquid cytology specimens to test for *C. trachomatis* and *N. gonorrhea*. Because NAATs detect DNA and RNA targets, they do not require viable organisms to detect infection. Therefore, if test of cure is needed, it should be delayed until all the chlamydial DNA/RNA has cleared, which usually takes more than 3 weeks.

The most common commercial test for *C. trachomatis* is the DNA probe, which uses nucleic acid hybridization to detect chlamydial DNA from urogenital swabs. The DNA probe detects an infection with specimens that have as few as 1,000 EBs. It has a sensitivity of 85–90 % and a specificity of 98–99 % compared to culture, and has a sensitivity of 77–93 % compared to NAATs [8]. Because the false positive rates with DNA probes are high, the CDC recommends that positive DNA probe test results in low-prevalence populations be confirmed by a second test [32]. One very attractive feature of the DNA probe is that the swab that is used to collect the specimen from the urogenital tract to test for *C. trachomatis* can also be used to test for *N. gonorrhea*.

Older non-culture diagnostic tests include direct fluorescent antibody (DFA) test and enzyme-linked immunoassay (EIA). DFA detects the outer membrane protein of EB and directly visualizes it with immunofluorescence. The sensitivity of DFA is only about 75 %, but it has a specificity of 98 %. At least ten EBs are necessary to detect infection. Clinical skills are required to obtain specimens. The sensitivity of DFA is often reduced by blood on the sample. Today, DFA is used most frequently in the laboratory to confirm positive results of other non-culture tests.

One of the earliest non-culture tests developed was EIA. EIA detects a chlamydia lipoprotein antigen by attaching specific antibodies coupled with an enzyme to the antibody. A color change occurs when the enzyme, which remains after binding with the antibody, acts upon a substrate. It takes approximately 10,000 EBs to cause an EIA to turn positive. The EIA has a sensitivity that varies from 62 to 75 % and has a specificity of 97 %. A major drawback of the older EIAs was that they bound to other gram negative organisms as well as *C. trachomatis*, which led to false positive test results. This problem has been overcome in newer versions by the addition of blocking reagents or by using DFA tests to confirm EIA results. When either of these additional methods is used, specificity is increased to 99 %. The antigen detection techniques are generally less expensive and easier to perform than NAATs. However, the antigen detection techniques have a lower sensitivity than NAATs, and they have lower positive predictive values. Therefore, if an antigen detection tests are used to screen a population with a 2–3 % prevalence of infection, about half of the results will return false positive (an incorrect result). For this reason, routine confirmation is generally recommended for positive cases.

Table 3.2 Recommendations for test selection for common chlamydia infection [32]

Endocervical swabs/urethral swabs	
Indication for testing	Test selection
• Screening	• Nucleic acid amplification tests (NAATs)
◆ Females: When pelvic examination is indicated	◆ Preferred because of high sensitivity relative to other tests
◆ Males: Urine might be more acceptable to asymptomatic males	• Non-culture/non-NAAT
• Endocervicitis	◆ Recommended when a NAAT is not available or not economical
• Urethritis (males)	• Culture
• Diseases at other anatomic locations possibly caused by sexually acquired *C. trachomatis* infection	◆ Preferred when an isolate is needed (e.g., sexual abuse or treatment failure)
◆ Pelvic inflammatory disease	• Point-of-care tests
◆ Urethral syndrome	◆ Recommended only when the patient is likely to be lost to follow-up and when the test will be performed while the patient waits for results and possible treatment
◆ Bartholinitis	• Additional testing is recommended after an initial positive screening test if a low positive predictive value can be expected or if a false positive result would have serious psychosocial or legal consequences
◆ Epididymitis	
◆ Perihepatitis (Fitz-Hugh-Curtis syndrome) (females)	
◆ Proctitis	
◆ Reactive arthritis/Reiter's syndrome	
◆ Conjunctivitis	
• Not recommended for prepubertal children	
Urethral swabs from women	
Indication for testing	Test selection
• Used with endocervical swab to increase sensitivity of culture for screening	• Culture
• Urethral syndrome	• Non-culture tests are not recommended

(continued)

Table 3.2 (continued)

Urine

Indication for testing

- Females: Screening or testing
- Males: Screening

Test selection

- NAAT
  - Recommended on the basis of increased sensitivity and ease of use
  - For males, sensitivity with urine has been lower than with urethral swab in the majority of studies, but not all
  - Other tests are not recommended because of low sensitivity and, in the case of enzyme immunoassay (EIA) and lipopolysaccharide (LPS)-specific direct fluorescent antibody (DFA) tests, lower specificity
  - Additional testing is recommended after an initial positive screening test if a low positive predictive value can be expected or if a false positive result would have serious psychosocial or legal consequences

Rectal swabs

Indication for testing

- Patients with history of receptive anal intercourse
- Proctitis
- Possible sexual abuse, children

Test selection

- Culture
  - Preferred when an isolate is needed (e.g., sexual abuse)
  - Sensitivity not well-defined; high specificity, especially if C. trachomatis-specific stain is used
  - Not readily available in most labs
- DFA
  - FDA-cleared for use with rectal specimens
  - Limited evaluation in published studies
  - Sensitivity not well-defined; potentially high specificity if *C. trachomatis*-specific stain is used
  - Other tests are not recommended
- NAAT
  - Although cross-reactivity with other rectal bacteria has not been reported for NAATs, they have received only limited evaluation in published studies
  - Some noncommercial labs have initiate NAATs that meet CLIA standards

Pharyngeal swabs

Indication for testing	Indication for testing

• Patients concerned regarding exposure during fellatio or cunnilingus
• Newborns or infants (nasopharyngeal specimens)
  ◆ Neonatal conjunctivitis
  ◆ Pneumonia consistent with *C. trachomatis* etiology
• Possible sexual abuse, children
	• Culture
	  ◆ Preferred method
	  ◆ Necessary when an isolate is needed (e.g., sexual abuse)
	  ◆ Sensitivity not well-defined; high specificity, including if *C. trachomatis*-specific stain is used
	• DFA
	  ◆ FDA-cleared for use with pharyngeal specimens
	  ◆ Limited evaluation in published studies
	  ◆ Sensitivity not well-defined; potentially high specificity if *C. trachomatis*-specific stain is used
	• Other tests are not recommended
	  ◆ NAAT
	    ■ Although cross-reactivity with other pharyngeal bacteria has not been reported for NAATs, they have received only limited evaluation in published studies

Conjunctivae swabs

Indication for testing	Test selection

• Conjunctivitis among adults
• Newborns or infants
  ◆ Neonatal conjunctivitis
  ◆ Pneumonia consistent with *C. trachomatis* etiology
	• Culture
	  ◆ Preferred, when available, because of high sensitivity and specificity
	• EIA, nucleic acid probe, and DFA tests
	  ◆ EIA, nucleic acid probe, and DFA tests that are FDA-cleared for use with conjunctival specimens have had uniformly high sensitivities with conjunctival specimens from newborns; evaluation studies are more limited for conjunctival specimens from adults with conjunctivitis
	  ◆ Specificities of tests on conjunctival specimens have also been high,†† although the potential for cross-reaction with other bacteria exists for EIA and for culture and DFA if used with stains that are not specific for *C. trachomatis*
	• Other tests are not recommended

Chlamydial infections can also be diagnosed by culture. The specimen must be cultured in tissue culture because *C. trachomatis* is an obligate intracellular organism and, therefore, is unable to grow on artificial media. Culture allows for antibiotic sensitivity testing as well as genotyping, which may be important for public health reasons. In the past, the sensitivity of culture techniques was thought to be close to 100 %. As a result, for many years, the culture was considered the gold standard. Today, however, it is recognized that at least 10–100 organisms are needed to result in a positive culture, but far fewer organisms can be detected by NAATs. Overall, it has been estimated that culture techniques have 65–85 % sensitivity compared to NAATs. The cost of tissue culture is higher than NAATs and it is technically difficult, labor intensive, and takes longer for results. However, in many courts, only the result of tissue culture may be introduced as evidence. The United States Drug and Food Administration (FDA) has not approved NAATs for the detection of pharyngeal and rectal chlamydial infections. In studies of MSM in whom detection rates of pharyngeal and rectal chlamydial infections by culture and NAATs were compared, the NAAT's tests showed twice the detection rate as compared with culture [33]. Future larger studies will be required to confirm these findings and the recommendation that NAATs be utilized in testing of these nongenital areas.

Regardless of the exact technology used to test for *C. trachomatis*, good specimen collection techniques are essential. In order to best detect the presence of *C. trachomatis*, infected cells should be collected. The scrapings from the endocervical area or the urethra are more apt to lead to detection of an infection than testing discharge. Using a cytobrush to collect cervical specimens improves the sensitivity of the culture and antigen detection tests. The cytobrush can safely be used in pregnant women to collect specimens. When urine specimens are to be tested, sensitivity is acceptable only if the first drops of urine are collected, without significant dilution from additional urine. The patient should not have urinated for at least 1 h prior to providing the specimen.

Antibodies for *C. trachomatis* can be assayed in serum. Serology for chlamydial antibodies is not useful in detection of acute infection because of poor specificity and reproducibility. In addition, serology and direct evidence of infection are not well correlated [34]. Therefore, serology cannot distinguish between active vs. resolved infection. Serology may be helpful in assessing if possible tubal factors are a cause of a woman's infertility and help determine who might benefit from hysterosalpingography [35].

Screening Recommendations

Targeted screening protocols are needed to control chlamydial infections for several reasons: the prevalence of *C. trachomatis* is relatively high, only a minority of women with chlamydial infections develops symptoms, and the sequellae of infection are potentially serious.

Routine screening of all sexually active women age 25 or younger is recommended whether or not the woman is pregnant. The frequency of subsequent testing of women under age 26 who are stable in mutually monogamous relationships after an initial negative test has not been determined. Screening of older women (>25) should be done only if these women are at increased risk (new or multiple sex partners, a prior history of a sexually transmitted infection, and inconsistent use of condoms in high risk relationships). The literature confirms the value of the routine screening of the sexually active females, 25 years or younger [36].

Routine screening of heterosexual men is not recommended, but testing is recommended for symptomatic men and those who are in setting with high prevalence of chlamydia (e.g., adolescent clinics, correctional facilities, and STD clinics). For sexually active MSM, the CDC recommends annual urethral/urine screening for chlamydia and rectal chlamydial cultures for MSM who have receptive anal sex. The CDC recommends screening every 3–6 months for MSM at highest risk (those with multiple sexual partners, or those who use illicit drugs) [20]. Men who are sex partners of infected women or men do not require testing for chlamydia infection prior to initiation of therapy, but might benefit from testing for public health reasons.

It is important to note that screening in low prevalence populations produces high false positive test results. The positive predictive value using a DNA probe test, performed in a setting with a prevalence of 2 %, is under 50 %. Because over half of the positive test results are not true positives (the patient is not infected with *C. trachomatis*), a confirmatory test is required. This can be done either by retesting the original specimen automatically in the laboratory or by performing a second test from the same or a different site in the patient.

Diagnosis

Clinical syndromes, such as nongonococcal urethritis or mucopurulent cervicitis may be diagnosed based on clinical signs and symptoms if supported by microscopic findings of leukocytosis. However, chlamydial infections are often asymptomatic, so diagnosis generally requires chlamydia-specific laboratory test identification/confirmation. Care must be taken, particularly in low risk patients and patients in low prevalence populations, to confirm positive test results to reduce the risk of false positivity.

In the face of laboratory-confirmed diagnosis of chlamydial cervicitis or urethritis, the patient should be evaluated for associated STIs. About 30 % of women with chlamydial cervicitis have concomitant trichomonal vaginitis. Gonorrhea accompanies chlamydial infections, but due to relatively low population prevalence, treatment for GC should await laboratory confirmation in most geographic areas. Other STIs, such as HIV, hepatitis B virus, and syphilis, should be evaluated on the basis of local prevalence rates.

Treatment

Because of the unique intracellular characteristics of *C. trachomatis*, only certain antibiotics are effective in treatment. The CDC treatment guidelines for chlamydial infections are summarized in Table 3.3 [20]. Tetracycline and doxycycline inhibit bacterial protein synthesis by blocking the attachment of the transfer RNA-amino acid to the ribosome. Common alternatives to doxycycline are the macrolide antibiotics, erythromycin or azithromycin. Macrolide antibiotics inhibit protein synthesis by binding to the p site on 50S RNA molecule of the bacterial ribosome, blocking the exit of the growing peptide chain. Azithromycin has high tissue penetration levels and a very long half-life, allowing a single dosing regimen. This enhances compliance and treatment success rates. Clinical cure rates for doxycycline and azithromycin are 96–99 % and 97 %, respectively [37, 38]. Resistance to tetracycline and macrolide antibiotics has been reported [39]. Single dose therapy with azithromycin is generally preferred because it is recognized that multiple dose therapies are often not completed. In one study of patients prescribed 7-day therapies with doxycycline, only 25 % of patients followed instructions completely, 24 % took no drug, and the remaining 51 % used some intermediate amount of the drug [40].

Table 3.3 Chlamydial Infection—CDC STD treatment guidelines 2010 [4]

Recommended regimens	Alternative regimens
Adolescents and adults. Select one of the following	
Azithromycin 1 g orally once	Erythromycin base 500 mg orally 4 times a day for 7 days
	Erythromycin ethylsuccinate 800 mg orally 4 times a day for 7 days
Doxycycline 100 mg orally twice a day for 7 days	Levofloxacin 500 mg orally daily for 7 days
	Ofloxacin 300 mg orally twice a day for 7 days
Pregnant women. Select one of the following	
Azithromycin 1 g orally once	Erythromycin base 500 mg orally 4 times a day for 7 days
	Erythromycin base 250 mg orally 4 times a day for 14 days
Amoxicillin 500 mg orally 3 times a day for 7 days	Erythromycin ethylsuccinate 800 mg orally 4 times a day for 7 days
	Erythromycin ethylsuccinate 400 mg orally 4 times a day for 14 days
Ophthalmia neonatorum caused by C. trachomatis	
Erythromycin base or ethylsuccinate 50 mg/kg/day orally divided into four doses daily for 14 days	
Chlamydial infections among children who weigh ≤45 kg	
Erythromycin base or ethylsuccinate 50 mg/kg/day orally divided into four doses daily for 14 days	
Chlamydial infections among children who weigh ≥45 kg but who are aged <8 years	
Azithromycin 1 g orally once	
Chlamydial infections among children aged ≥8 years. Select one of the following	
Azithromycin 1 g orally once	
Doxycycline 100 mg orally twice a day for 7 days	

Quinolone antibiotics act by targeting two enzymes, DNA gyrase and topoisomerase IV, which are necessary for DNA replication. Within this group of antibiotics, ofloxacin and levofloxacin are most effective. *C. trachomatis* has the potential to mutate leading to quinolone resistance when exposed to subinhibitory concentrations of antibiotics [41]. Patients should be encouraged to complete all medications for their full course of therapy.

Amoxicillin has similar efficacy to erythromycin, with less side effects, and can be used in pregnancy when the patient cannot tolerate erythromycin. Other penicillin and all cephalosporin antibiotics have no role in the management of chlamydial infections [42].

Patients should be instructed to abstain from all sexual contact until all of their sex partners have been treated. Treatment is considered complete 7 days after finishing medication. The need for this counseling was highlighted by a study of 597 college women randomized to azithromycin vs. doxycycline in which two pregnancies occurred during the 2-week study period [38]. Patients should also be counseled on future consistent use of condoms and other safer sex practices.

Follow-up

It is not necessary to perform a routine test of cure after therapy, except in women treated with erythromycin. It is recognized that erythromycin causes many side effects and that compliance is therefore often poor. Repeat testing of all nonpregnant women with chlamydial infection should be considered 3 months after treatment. This is particularly important for adolescent women who often return to the same high risk environment from which they acquired their first infections. Routine repeat testing is also encouraged at every other examination done 3–12 months after treatment regardless of whether the patient believes that her sex partner(s) was treated.

Complications of Infection

Infertility, ectopic pregnancy and pelvic pain are sequellae of both symptomatic and asymptomatic PID. In women with confirmed PID, infertility was seen in 16 % vs. 2.7 % of controls. Ectopic pregnancy was 9.1 % vs. 1.4 % and tubal factor infertility was 10.8 % vs. 0 % [43]. The risk of infertility increases with number of episodes and severity of the inflammation. In women who had had PID, hospital readmissions for abdominal and pelvic pain were significantly more likely and the risk for hysterectomy was 6 times greater than controls [44]. Chronic pelvic pain after PID is associated with reduced physical and mental health [45].

Partner Notification and Reporting Requirements

Chlamydia is a reportable disease in all 50 states. All sexual contacts for the 60 days prior to onset of symptoms (or diagnosis of asymptomatic infections) should be evaluated, tested, and treated. It is important to note that it is not necessary to await positive test results for chlamydial infection to initiate partner therapy; therapy for chlamydial infection should be given to partners on an epidemiologic basis. Treatment for other possible STIs not detected in the index case should await laboratory confirmation.

If there is concern that a heterosexual sex partner will not seek care, the CDC suggests that the patient can provide the partner the treatment. In California, state law allows clinicians to treat sex partners of patients found to have laboratory-confirmed genital chlamydial infections without co-infection with gonorrhea or other complications. Under this law, treatment for chlamydia can be given without any contact or evaluation, even if the partner is not a patient of the clinician. This provision (patient-delivered partner therapy) is generally reserved for partners who are not expected not to seek care for the problem. The recommended treatment is azithromycin. Specialized instructions that explain the reason for the treatment and screen for macrolide allergy (e.g., erythromycin) accompany the medications. Also included in the packet is encouragement to seek professional care to be evaluated for other (as yet undiagnosed) STIs. Recently, research has demonstrated again that expedited treatment with patient-delivered partner therapy reduced the rates of persistent or recurrent gonorrhea and chlamydial infection but gonorrhea reduction was more significant than chlamydia reduction [46]. Patient-delivered partner therapy is not recommended for MSM because of the high risk of coexisting infections in that partner, especially HIV.

Special Pregnancy-Related Issues

The association between chlamydial cervicitis and preterm rupture of membranes, preterm labor and preterm delivery has been strongly suggested by two clinical trials, which served as a basis for CDC recommendation for screening in pregnancy [47, 48]. However, no prospective placebo-controlled studies have verified this association. Given the strength of the association found in these earlier studies, however, it may not be ethical to conduct placebo-controlled trials. The role *C. trachomatis* plays in the etiology of postpartum endometritis is controversial, but the diagnosis should be considered when women present 2–3 weeks postpartum with fever, chills, purulent lochia, and a tender, boggy, enlarged uterus. Women infected with *C. trachomatis* at delivery were more likely to experience febrile complications after postpartum tubal ligation [49]. The association of chlamydial cervicitis and postabortal infection is clear. Estimates are that 10–35 % of women who undergo elective abortion with chlamydial cervicitis will develop postabortal endometritis/PID. This observation has led to the practice of routine antibiotic prophylaxis at the time of surgical abortion.

In pregnancy, the optimal testing scheduled has not been established but the CDC recommend testing prenatal patient under 26 and other high-risk women depending on local prevalence rates. Early testing could reduce pregnancy risks associated with infection, such as low birth weight and premature delivery. Testing late in pregnancy can decrease transmission to the infant and diminish the risk of postpartum maternal infections. Combined testing has not been evaluated.

Doxycycline should not be used in pregnancy. In pregnant women, test of cure is routinely recommended by the CDC, although some experts do not deem it necessary if the patient was treated with azithromycin. It is important to wait 3 weeks from the completion of therapy to do test of cure, since some tests may detect *C. trachomatis* remnants even after the organisms have been eradicated. Infected women should be retested in the third trimester.

Prevention

A National Institute of Health (NIH) panel performed a comprehensive review of the literature in 2000 and concluded that there was not sufficient evidence to allow an accurate assessment of the degree of protection against chlamydia offered by correct and consistent condom use (see Chapter on Barriers) [50]. The CDC recommends condom use to reduce the spread of chlamydia [51]. A recent study with a case-crossover design suggested that correct and consistent condom use was associated with a 50 % reduction in chlamydial infection. The investigators were also able to identify a dose–response relationship. In 2004, a review of studies published after the NIH conference found that the literature in that time period supported the conclusion that condom use was associated with statistically significant protection for men and women form chlamydia infection [52]. An analysis of 45 studies published between 1966 and 2004 concluded that most studies found that condom use was associated with a reduced risk of chlamydia in both men and women [53].

References

1. Centers for Disease Control and Prevention. Sexually transmitted diseases surveillance. Atlanta, GA: Centers for Disease Control and Prevention; 2010. Available from: http://www.cdc.gov/std/stats10/surv2010.pdf.
2. Chesson HW, Blandford JM, Gift TL, et al. The estimated direct medical cost of sexually transmitted diseases among American youth, 2000. Perspect Sex Reprod Health. 2004;36(1):11–9.
3. Weinstock H, Berman S, Cates Jr W. Sexually transmitted diseases among American youth: incidence and prevalence estimates, 2000. Perspect Sex Reprod Health. 2004;36:6–10.
4. Centers for Disease Control and Prevention. Sexually transmitted diseases treatment guidelines, 2010. MMWR. 2010;59(RR-12):9.

5. Turner CF, Rogers SM, Miller HG, et al. Untreated gonococcal and chlamydia infection in a probability sample of adults. JAMA. 2002;287:726–33.
6. Groseclose SL, Zaidi AA, DeLisle SJ, et al. Estimated incidence and prevalence of genital Chlamydia trachomatis infections in the United States, 1996. Sex Transm Dis. 1999; 26(6):339–44.
7. World Health Organization. Prevalence and incidence of selected sexually transmitted infections. Geneva: World Health Organization; 2011.
8. Sweet RL, Gibbs RS. Chlamydial infections. In: Sweet RL, Gibbs RS, editors. Infectious diseases of the female genital tract. 4th ed. Philadelphia: Lippincott Williams & Wilkins; 2002. p. 57–100.
9. Miller WC, Ford CA, Morris M, et al. Prevalence of chlamydial and gonococcal infections among young adults in the United States. JAMA. 2004;291(18):2229–36.
10. Kent CK, Chaw JK, Wong W, et al. Prevalence of rectal, utrethral, and pharyngeal chlamydia and gonorrhea detected in 2 clinical setting among men who have sex with men: San Francisco, California, 2003. Clin Infect Dis. 2005;41:67–74.
11. Mimiaga MJ, Mayer KH, Reisner SL, et al. Asymptomatic gonorrhea and chlamydial infections detected by nucleic acid amplification tests among Boston area men who have sex with men. Sex Transm Dis. 2008;35:495.
12. Forward KR. Risk of coinfection with Chlamydia trachomatis and Neisseria gonorrhoeae in Nova Scotia. Can J Infect Dis Med Microbiol. 2010;21(2):e84–6.
13. Jacobson DL, Peralta L, Graham NM, Zenilman J. Histologic development of cervical ectopy: relationship to reproductive hormones. Sex Transm Dis. 2000;27(5):252–8.
14. Quinn TC, Gaydos C, Shepherd M, Bobo L, et al. Epidemiologic and microbiologic correlates of Chlamydia trachomatis infection in sexual partnerships. JAMA. 1996;276(21):1737–42.
15. Morre SA, Rozendaal L, van Valkengoed IG, et al. Urogenital Chlamydia trachomatis serovars in men and women with a symptomatic or asymptomatic infection: an association with clinical manifestations? J Clin Microbiol. 2000;38(6):2292–6.
16. Davies JA, Rees E, Hobson D, Karayiannis P. Isolation of Chlamydia trachomatis from Bartholin's ducts. Br J Vener Dis. 1978;54(6):409–13.
17. Saul HM, Grossman MB. The role of Chlamydia trachomatis in Bartholin's gland abscess. Am J Obstet Gynecol. 1988;158(3 Pt 1):76–7.
18. Bleker OP, Smalbraak DJ, Schutte MF. Bartholin's abscess: the role of Chlamydia trachomatis. Genitourin Med. 1990;66(1):24–5.
19. Batteiger BE, Jones RB. Chlamydial infections. Infect Dis Clin North Am. 1987;1(1):55–81.
20. Workowski KA, Berman S, Centers for Disease Control and Prevention (CDC). Sexually transmitted diseases treatment guidelines, 2010. MMWR Recomm Rep. 2010;59:1.
21. Mutlu N, Mutlu B, Culha M, et al. The role of Chlamydia trachomatis in patients with nonbacterial prostatitis. Int J Clin Pract. 1998;52(8):540–1.
22. Ostaszewska I, Zdrodowska-Stefanow B, Badyda J, et al. Chlamydia trachomatis: probable cause of prostatitis. Int J STD AIDS. 1998;9(6):350–3.
23. Ness RB, Markovic N, Carlson CL, Coughlin MT. Do men become infertile after having sexually transmitted urethritis? An epidemiologic examination. Fertil Steril. 1997;68(2):205–13.
24. Thompson CI, MacAulay AJ, Smith IW. Chlamydia trachomatis infections in the female rectums. Genitourin Med. 1989;65(4):269–73.
25. Wexner SD. Sexually transmitted diseases of the colon, rectum, and anus. The challenge of the nineties. Dis Colon Rectum. 1990;33(12):1048–62.
26. Silveira LH, Gutierrez F, Scopelitis E, et al. Chlamydia-induced reactive arthritis. Rheum Dis Clin North Am. 1993;19(2):351–62.
27. Hanada H, Ikeda-Dantsuji Y, Naito M, Nagayama A. Infection of human fibroblast-like synovial cells with Chlamydia trachomatis results in persistent infection and interleukin-6 production. Microb Pathog. 2003;34(2):57–63.
28. Schachter J, Grossman M, Sweet RL, et al. Prospective study of perinatal transmission of Chlamydia trachomatis. JAMA. 1986;255(24):3374–7.

29. Bell TA, Stamm WE, Kuo CC, et al. Risk of perinatal transmission of Chlamydia trachomatis by mode of delivery. J Infect. 1994;29(2):165–9.
30. Jain S. Perinatally acquired Chlamydia trachomatis associated morbidity in young infants. J Matern Fetal Med. 1999;8(3):130–3.
31. Weiss SG, Newcomb RW, Beem MO. Pulmonary assessment of children after chlamydial pneumonia of infancy. J Pediatr. 1986;108(5 Pt 1):659–64.
32. Johnson RE, Newhall WJ, Papp JR, et al. Screening tests to detect Chlamydia trachomatis and Neisseria gonorrhoeae infections—2002. MMWR Recomm Rep. 2002;51(RR-15):1–38.
33. Schachter J, Moncada J, Liska S, et al. Nucleic acid amplification tests in the diagnosis of chlamydial and gonococcal infections of the oropharynx and rectum in men who have sex with men. Sex Transm Dis. 2008;35:637.
34. Rabenau HF, Kohler E, Peters M, et al. Low correlation of serology with detection of Chlamydia trachomatis by ligase chain reaction and antigen EIA. Infection. 2000;28(2):97–102.
35. Akande VA, Hunt LP, Cahill DJ, et al. Tubal damage in infertile women: prediction using chlamydia serology. Hum Reprod. 2003;18(9):1841–7.
36. U.S. Preventive Services Task Force. Screening for chlamydial infection: U.S. Preventive Services Task Force recommendation statement. Ann Intern Med. 2007;147:128.
37. Martin DH, Mroczkowski TF, Dalu ZA, et al. A controlled trial of a single dose of azithromycin for the treatment of chlamydial urethritis and cervicitis. The Azithromycin for Chlamydial Infections Study Group. N Engl J Med. 1992;327(13):921–5.
38. Thorpe Jr EM, Stamm WE, Hook III EW, Gall SA, Jones RB, Henry K, et al. Chlamydial cervicitis and urethritis: single dose treatment compared with doxycycline for seven days in community based practices. Genitourin Med. 1996;72(2):93–7.
39. Somani J, Bhullar VB, Workowski KA, et al. Multiple drug-resistant Chlamydia trachomatis associated with clinical treatment failure. J Infect Dis. 2000;181(4):1421–7.
40. Augenbraun M, Bachmann L, Wallace T, et al. Compliance with doxycycline therapy in sexually transmitted diseases clinics. Sex Transm Dis. 1998;25(1):1–4.
41. Silverman NS, Sullivan M, Hochman M, et al. A randomized, prospective trial comparing amoxicillin and erythromycin for the treatment of Chlamydia trachomatis in pregnancy. Am J Obstet Gynecol. 1994;170(3):829–32.
42. Ridgway GL. Treatment of chlamydial genital infection. J Antimicrob Chemother. 1997;40(3):311–4.
43. Westrom L, Joesoef R, Reynolds G, et al. Pelvic inflammatory disease and fertility. A cohort study of 1,844 women with laparoscopically verified disease and 657 control women with normal laparoscopic result. Sex Transm Dis. 1992;19:185–92.
44. Buchan H, Vessey M, Goldacre M, Fairweather J. Morbidity following pelvic inflammatory disease. Br J Obstet Gynaecol. 1993;100:558–62.
45. Haggerty CL, Schulz R, Ness RB, PID Evaluation and Clinical Health Study Investigators. Lower quality of life among women with chronic pelvic pain after pelvic inflammatory disease. Obstet Gynecol. 2003;102:934–9.
46. Golden MR, Whittington WL, Handsfield HH, et al. Effect of expedited treatment of sex partners on recurrent or persistent gonorrhea or chlamydial infection. N Engl J Med. 2005;352(7):676–85.
47. Ryan Jr GM, Abdella TN, McNeeley SG, et al. Chlamydia trachomatis infection in pregnancy and effect of treatment on outcome. Am J Obstet Gynecol. 1990;162(1):34–9.
48. Cohen I, Veille JC, Calkins BM. Improved pregnancy outcome following successful treatment of chlamydial infection. JAMA. 1990;263(23):3160–3.
49. Todd CS, Jones RB, Golichowski A, Arno JN. Chlamydia trachomatis and febrile complications of postpartum tubal ligation. Am J Obstet Gyncol. 1997;176:100–2.
50. National Institute of Allergy and Infectious Disease. Workshop summary. Scientific evidence on condom effectiveness for sexually transmitted disease (STD) prevention. National Institutes of Health, Department of Health and Human Services; 2001. Available from: http://www.niaid.nih.gov/about/organization/dmid/Documents/condomreport.pdf.

51. Centers for Disease Control and Prevention. Condoms and STDs: fact sheet for public health personnel, National Center for HIV, STD and TB Prevention; 2011. Available from: www.cdc.gov/condomeffectiveness/latex.htm.
52. Holmes KK, Levine R, Weaver M. Effectiveness of condoms in preventing sexually transmitted infections. Bull World Health Organ. 2004;82:454–61.
53. Warner L, Stone KM, Macaluso M, et al. Condom use and risk of gonorrhea and chlamydia: a systematic review of design and measurement factors assessed in epidemiologic studies. Sex Transm Dis. 2006;33:36–51.

Chapter 4
Gonorrhea

Jennifer E. Thuener and Amy Lynn Clouse

Introduction

Gonorrhea has been a public nuisance long before it was identified as a bacterium. Gonorrhea can be identified as one of the oldest known human diseases. References to a urethritis acquired from sexual contact can be read about in the Old Testament, and ancient Chinese writings [1]. Its name is quite descriptive of its symptoms, as least in men. The name gonorrhea, is derived of "flow of seed," was coined in 130 AD when it was noted that the purulent discharge of this disease appeared similar to semen. Not until as recently as 1879 was German physician Albert Neisser able to identify and describe the bacteria causing such nuisance, *Neisseria gonorrhoeae* [1]. Despite a known cause, physicians had no true treatment for gonorrhea until the 1930s brought the advent of antibiotics; first with sulfonamides then penicillin in the 1940s. However, *N. gonorrhoeae* has continued to be a troublesome bug, growing resistant to multiple treatments, including penicillin. The medical community today must remain continuously vigilant, and stay ahead of resistance of this hardy and common bacterium.

J.E. Thuener, MD (✉)
Family Medicine, Abington Memorial Hospital, 500 Old York Road,
Suite 108, Jenkintown, PA 19046, USA
e-mail: Jennifer.thuener.md@gmail.com

A.L. Clouse, MD
Abington Family Medicine, Abington Memorial Hospital, Jenkintown, PA 19046, USA

N.S. Skolnik et al. (eds.), *Sexually Transmitted Diseases: A Practical Guide for Primary Care*, Current Clinical Practice, DOI 10.1007/978-1-62703-499-9_4,
© Springer Science+Business Media New York 2013

Prevalence/Incidence

Gonorrhea is a common infectious disease. In the United States alone there are around 700,000 new *N. gonorrhoeae* infections each year [2]. The actual reported cases remain around 300,000 per year; however, officials believe that the number of infections is so significantly underreported, that the true numbers are double the reported estimate [1]. Most cases occur in sexually active 15–24-year-old women, with the highest rate among women aged 15–19 according to 2010 data, accounting for 570.9 cases per 100,000 [2]. The Centers for Disease Control and Prevention (CDC) also has consistently found that the rate of gonorrhea infection in minorities, specifically black Americans, is far greater than the rate of infection in white Americans [3]. The rate of gonorrhea among blacks was 432.5 per 100,000, which is 18.7 times higher than among whites [3].

Men who have sex with men (MSM) likely have higher rates of gonorrhea than any other population. National data from the CDC is not available; however, the King County, Washington health department estimated the rate of gonorrhea among MSM to be 719 per 100,000, and the CDC does note that 15 % of MSM who report to surveillance STD clinics were positive for gonorrhea. HIV positive men are also more likely to have gonorrhea than their HIV negative counterparts, possibly due to increased risky sexual activity [4].

Risk Factors

The prevalence of gonorrhea varies drastically from community to community, so when determining potential risk factors of a given patient population, one should take into account the prevalence of gonorrhea within the community. The risk factor that consistently lends itself to higher rates of gonorrhea is younger age—likely due to increased sexual partners and less consistent condom use [5]. As previously mentioned, having HIV also is a risk factor, likely due to tendency towards riskier sexual behaviors. Furthermore, HIV can make one more susceptible to gonorrhea infection and more likely to transmit the bacteria to other individuals.

Infectivity and Transmission

Gonorrhea is passed from one partner to another almost exclusively through sexual contact. Gonorrhea is readily passed from genital to genital through contact, but is less transmissible from mouth to genital or vice versa. Transmission through anal sex has been reported as well, although the exact rates are not as well studied. The risk of transmission from an infected female to a male is about 20 % per unprotected episode of vaginal intercourse, and increases after 4 or more exposures to 60–80 %. Transmission rates from an infected male to female by vaginal intercourse are much higher at an estimated 70 % per episode of unprotected sex [1].

Transmission of gonorrhea is concerning, not only because of the morbidity of the gonorrhea bacteria, but because current infection with gonorrhea can increase one's susceptibility to HIV in a noninfected person, and increase transmission of HIV in an infected person [2].

A neonate delivered from a woman with active gonorrhea cervicitis has a 30–35 % risk of contracting gonococcal conjunctivitis. Due to routine prophylaxis with antibiotic ointment in infants shortly after birth, neonatal conjunctival infection in America is now rare [6].

Gonorrhea has a relatively short incubation period, typically less than 2 weeks in women and 2–3 days in men. As a direct result, men tend to seek earlier treatment, while woman can remain infected without symptoms for longer, leading females to be the more frequent transmitters of the disease [1].

Etiology

Neisseria gonorrhoeae, a gram negative coccus typically grows in pairs, commonly called diplococci. While all Neisseria species have fastidious culture requirements, *Neisseria* is a nitrate reducer, and can only reduce glucose, causing it to require specific agar necessary for growth. Neisseria is typically grown on Thayer Martin plate, which is a chocolate agar with antibiotics that will inhibit the growth of other organisms [1].

Gonococci are not very tolerant of dry conditions, which may explain why fomite transmission of gonorrhea is nearly nonexistent. While Gonococci are nonmotile, they do have pili attached to the outer wall. Gonococci are also noted to have a strong preference to columnar or cuboidal epithelium. This gives a clear insight into the increased ease of transmission of gonococci to the genitourinary tract, where columnar and cuboidal cells predominate [1].

N. gonorrhoeae's main method of infectivity is through adherence to the host's epithelial cell, so those bacteria with stronger pili are more virulent than those without pili. Some of the body's own mechanisms keep gonococci at bay as *Lactobacillus jensenii*, a typical component of healthy vaginal flora, reduces the ability of gonococci to adhere to the epithelium. This likely plays a large part in the observation that bacterial vaginitis, which involves a loss of these healthy bacteria, places a person at an increased risk of gonococcal infection [1].

Clinical Manifestations

Women

Gonorrhea is most easily transmitted via penile—vaginal intercourse. In women, the most common place of infection is the cervix. *N. Gonorrhoeae* is most attracted to columnar epithelium, and therefore will preferentially infect the endocervix.

Over 95 % of infected woman are asymptomatic; however, if symptoms are present, they commonly include dyspareunia, postcoital bleeding, and vaginal discharge [7]. On clinical exam, the most common findings are purulent cervical discharge and a friable cervix. Women that develop symptoms generally do so within 10 days of infection. Since more than half of infected women are asymptomatic, there is a fairly high rate of ascending infection extending into the endometrium and fallopian tubes [7]. This infection, commonly known as pelvic inflammatory disease (PID) will develop in 10–20% of woman infected with gonorrhea [7]. Fallopian tube scarring is a relatively common complication and up to 15 % of women have problems with fertility after just one episode of PID. After three episodes of PID, as many as 50 % of women are infertile [8].

Men

The most common sequelae of gonorrhea in men is urethritis. Men have a much shorter latent period, they will usually present with symptoms within 2–3 days of infection. Symptoms of urethritis typically consist of dysuria and penile discharge. Gonococcal discharge may start as scant and watery, but within 2 days it develops into the thick, purulent discharge that is typically associated with gonorrhea. If untreated, gonococcal urethritis will resolve spontaneously over a few weeks although the disease continues to be highly transmissible throughout this time [7].

Both Men and Women

Pharyngeal infection—gonorrhea can infect the mucosa of the throat, but this infection is rarely symptomatic. Transmission is most commonly from fellatio. Gonococcal pharyngitis is commonly a coinfection with gonorrhea at other sites, either genital or rectal. There is some data that screening women for gonorrhea of the throat will lead to a higher rate of diagnosis; however, there is uncertain significance of isolated pharyngeal gonorrhea infection, as symptoms are rare and spontaneous resolution is common. Transmission from an infected throat to a partner during oral sex is rare [1].

Rectal gonorrhea infection—rectal gonorrhea can be seen in both men and women. The importance of diagnosing rectal gonorrhea is unclear in women, as it is frequently coexisting with cervical gonorrhea; however, in MSM, it is often the only site of infection, making the diagnosis of rectal gonorrhea much more salient in this population. Rates of rectal transmission to a previously uninfected male are not known. While this infection is usually asymptomatic, it can cause an overt infection, with symptoms of tenesmus, anal pruritus, purulent discharge, or rectal bleeding [8].

Conjunctivitis

Gonorrhea can cause conjunctivitis in the newborn from gonorrhea acquired during birth. Rare cases of gonococcal conjunctivitis are seen in adults, and this is usually seen as a coinfection with rectal or genital gonorrhea. The conjunctivitis is typically painful with thick copious discharge, the infection can progress to cause corneal ulceration unless treated [1].

Neonatal conjunctivitis is now rare in the United States due to prophylactic eye drops in the neonatal period. It should be suspected when an acute conjunctivitis occurs shortly after birth, usually within 2–3 days [1].

Disseminated Infection

A rare complication of gonorrhea infection is disseminated gonococcal infection (DGI). This is reported to happen in 0.5–3 % of patients infected with gonorrhea. The most common manifestation of DGI is the arthritis-dermatitis syndrome, as 70 % of patients with DGI present with these symptoms [6]. This involves arthralgias involving multiple joints that tend to move from one joint to another. Skin lesions are often pustular or vesicular, painless, and involve the extremities. This initial presentation will often resolve, or can evolve into a septic arthritis, usually in a single joint. Any sexually active young adult with distal joint pain or suspicious skin lesions should be suspect for gonorrhea, and screened at any expose site. If left untreated, DGI will generally resolve; however, an overtly septic untreated joint may develop joint destruction or osteomyelitis [6].

Screening

The U.S. Preventive Services Task Force (USPSTF) currently recommends AGAINST screening for gonorrheal infection in low risk populations. Low risk groups are not clearly defined; however, we may assume this includes heterosexual patients over the age of 25 who do not engage in high risk activities. High risk behavior includes having multiple or new sexual partners, inconsistent condom use, or living in an area with high rate of infection. Other risk factors include low socio-economic status, recreational drug or alcohol use, or exchanging sex for drugs or money. The USPSTF notes that being under the age of 25 is the highest risk factor.

The CDC currently recommends screening MSM yearly based on their sexual activity. Men who have had insertive intercourse in the last year should have urethral or urine DNA testing for gonorrhea and chlamydia. Yearly screening for rectal gonorrhea and chlamydia infection is recommended for men who have had receptive anal intercourse in the past year. Likewise, yearly DNA swab or culture for pharyngeal infection is recommended for men who have had receptive oral intercourse in the past year. For MSM that are at very high risk, including those who have multiple or anonymous partners, screening should be considered every 3–6 months [2].

Testing and Diagnosis

There are currently three different categories of testing for gonorrhea. The first is direct visualization via gram stain, the second is a culture of the bacteria, and the third is by direct assessment of the genetic components of the bacteria, known as Nucleic Acid Amplification Tests, or NAATs. This can be accomplished by amplification of either DNA or RNA. Currently there are three types of NAATs available: polymerase chain reaction (PCR), strand displacement amplification (SDA), and transcription mediated amplification (TMA). Because of a high sensitivity and ease of testing, NAATs have now replaced the bacterial culture for diagnosis of gonorrhea infections [9]. However, NAATs are currently only FDA approved for male urethral, female cervical and urine specimens of men and women [9].

In symptomatic men, a gram stain that demonstrates gonorrhea can be considered diagnostic. A gram stain of urethral discharge has a specificity of greater than 99 % and a sensitivity of 95 %. Given this slightly lower sensitivity, a gram stain is not recommended for screening of an asymptomatic male, and is also not considered a good test for cervical, pharyngeal, or rectal specimens [10].

The gold standard for diagnosis of genital and ophthalmic gonorrhea is a bacterial culture. *Neisseria gonorrhoeae* is a difficult bacterium to culture, requiring a selective media, a CO_2-enriched environment, and incubation at 36 °C. A bacterial culture is also the only test that will give the practitioner data on antibiotic sensitivity, so in any case where treatment failure is suspected, it is vital that a culture be taken [1].

It may prove challenging to identify gonorrheal infection from pharyngeal and rectal samples. While culture of these regions is the only truly recommended and approved test, cultures have low sensitivity. Furthermore, there is not a true gold standard test for gonorrhea in these areas, leaving it very difficult to establish sensitivities and specificities of any tests of infection of the pharynx or rectum. There are also concerns of a false positive result from a pharyngeal culture as non-gonococcal *Neisseria* may be colonized [9].

Treatment

Treatment of gonorrheal infections has changed rapidly over the past decade as *N. gonorrhoeae* has become resistant to many antibiotics, including sulfonamides, penicillin, tetracyclines, macrolides, and fluoroquinolones. In light of the rapid resistance and the high prevalence of gonorrhea, the CDC established a program to monitor antibiotic resistance of *N. gonorrhoeae* in 1986 known as the Gonococcal Isolate Surveillance Project (GISP). The CDC collects culture data from the first 25 men to be diagnosed with gonorrhea in each of 28 clinics from different cities in the United States. These samples are then tested for resistance to penicillin, tetracycline, spectinomycin, ciprofloxacin, ceftriaxone, cefixime, and azithromycin [3]. With this data, the CDC is able to monitor resistance patterns and recommend appropriate changes in therapy. The most recent treatment change from GISP came in August 2012, updating the latest guidelines on the treatment of gonorrhea from the CDC that were published in 2010. At that time, the treatment regimen was Ceftriaxone 250 mg intramuscular (IM) once OR Cefixime 400 mg orally once. Alternatively, an oral cephlasporin PLUS azithromycin or doxycycline could have been used [2]. The CDC also recommended co-treatment with azithromycin or doxycycline, even if a negative chlamydia PCR is present [2]. Through the GISP data, there was concern for growing resistance to oral cefixime, and as of August 10, 2012, the CDC has published new treatment recommendations.

For all uncomplicated infections of gonorrhea of the cervix, urethra, pharynx, and rectum, the recommended treatment is ceftriaxone 250 mg intramuscular once PLUS either azithromycin 1 g orally in a single dose OR doxycycline 100 mg orally twice daily for 7 days. Of note, azithromycin is preferred over doxycycline in the CDC guidelines as it provides better coverage in conjunction with the ceftriaxone. The addition of azithromycin is for the treatment of gonorrhea as it covers nearly all isolates of gonorrhea, and will hopefully slow progression to resistance to ceftriaxone [11].

If intramuscular ceftriaxone is unavailable, there are two alternative regimens for treatment of urogenital or rectal gonorrhea: cefixime 400 mg in a single oral dose *PLUS*, azithromycin 1 g orally in a single dose, or doxycycline 100 mg orally twice a day for 7 days. If the patient has a life-threatening allergy to cephalosporins, then azithromycin 2 g in a single oral dose is recommended. There is no recommended alternative therapy for pharyngeal gonorrhea. All patients receiving any treatment other than the recommended regimen of ceftriaxone plus azithromycin need a test of cure of the infected site in 1 week either by culture or NAAT. Culture is recommended in these instances to check antimicrobial susceptibility testing [11].

Partner Treatment

All partners who have had sexual contact with the patient within the past 60 days should be treated for gonorrhea, whether or not symptoms are present. The current recommendation from the CDC is to have the patient direct all partners to a physician or clinic for screening and subsequent treatment. If the patient denies any sexual contact during the past 60 days, then the most recent sexual contact should be treated. Patients should be advised to refrain from sexual activity until both the patient and all current partners have been adequately treated and any symptoms have resolved to avoid reinfection [2].

In the past years, there has been a movement to treat partners of infected patients via expedited partner therapy, meaning that medication is dispensed to partners of infected patients without having the partners seen by a physician. This practice should only be used with heterosexual patients, as the risk of coinfection with HIV and syphilis is markedly increased in the homosexual population, as is the incidence of resistant gonorrhea. Partners of MSM who test positive for gonorrhea should be directed to seek treatment [11]. There have been no clear recommendations to using expedited partner therapy with the new guidelines that recommend against treating with oral cephalosporins; however, logic would suggest that expedited partner therapy may be a recommendation of the past, given the preferred treatment is with an intramuscular injection which requires the patient to seek care in a physician's office. Since management with one of the alternative antibiotics regimens requires a follow-up test of cure posttreatment, it may make more sense for patients' partners to seek treatment with a physician rather than via expedited therapy.

Follow up

Currently, the CDC does not have a recommendation for test of cure of gonorrhea, except as noted above in the case of suboptimal treatment, which includes any regimen other than the recommended ceftriaxone plus azithromycin. When any alternative therapy is used for the treatment of gonorrhea, including an oral cephalosporin or 2 g azithromycin, a test of cure is recommended 1 week after initial treatment [11].

There is also some evidence for rescreening a patient 3 months after the initial infection, not as a test of cure, but as a screen for reinfection. Patients who have been infected with gonorrhea have shown themselves to be in a higher risk group that the general population, and therefore, they are more likely to have a reinfection within 3 months [12]. Testing at 3 months should include not only testing for gonorrhea, but for other STDs as well, such as chlamydia, trichomonas, HIV, and syphilis, as they are in general at higher risk for all STDs [12].

Prevention

Counseling patients on safer sex is the most effective way to reduce rates of STDs in any population. As with any patient interaction, open communication in a non-judgmental way about safer sexual practices, such as using condoms with every partner, reducing the number of partners, and choosing partners carefully. A reliable method of reducing STD infections is abstaining from oral, anal, and vaginal sex or only having sex with one partner in a long-term relationship. Condom use can be protective; however, condoms need to be used in every sexual encounter, and used prior to first contact [2].

While counseling can be effective, physicians need to remember to counsel about safe sexual practices at every visit. The CDC recommends counseling patients specific to their situation, which involves asking the patient detailed questions about their current sexual practices, and then giving patient-specific advice on how to reduce their current risk factors. This approach has been found to reduce STD rates as well as risky sexual behaviors [2].

References

1. Mandell GL, Bennett E, Dolin R. Mandell, Douglas, and Bennett's principles and practice of infectious diseases. Orlando: Churchill Livingstone; 2009.
2. Centers for Disease Control and Prevention. Gonococcal infections. MMWR. 2010;17:49–55.
3. Centers for Disease Control and Prevention. Gonococcal Isolate Surveillance Project (GISP) [Internet]. 2012. Available from: http://www.cdc.gov/STD/gisp/default.htm.
4. Centers for Disease Control and Prevention. Cephalosporin susceptibility among Neisseria gonorrhoeae isolates—United States, 2000-2010. MMWR Wkly. 2011;60:873–7.
5. Hwang LSM. Chlamydia trachomatis infection in adolescents. Adv Pediatr. 2004;51:379–407.
6. Goldman L, Schafer A. Goldman's Cecil medicine. St. Louis: W.B. Saunders; 2011.
7. Miller K. Diagnosis and treatment of Nessieria gonorrhoeae infections. Am Fam Physician. 2006;15:1779–84.
8. Creighton S. Gonorrhea. Am Fam Physician. 2012;85(6):642–3.
9. Renault CA, Hall C, Kent CK, Klausner JD. Use of NAATs for STD diagnosis of GC and CT in non-FDA-cleared anatomic specimens. Med Lab Obs. 2006;38(7):10; 12–6; 21–2.
10. Mayor MT, Roett AM, Uduhiri KA. Diagnosis and management of gonococcal infections. Am Fam Physician. 2012;86(10):931–8.
11. Centers for Disease Control and Prevention. Update to CDC's sexually transmitted diseases treatment guidelines, 2010: oral cephalosporins no longer a recommended treatment for gonococcal infections. MMWR Wkly. 2012;61:590–4.
12. Peterman TA, Tian LH, Metcaf CA. High incidence of new sexually transmitted infections in the year following a sexually transmitted infection: a case for rescreening. Ann Intern Med. 2006;17:564–72.

Chapter 5
Pelvic Inflammatory Disease

Joshua H. Barash, Christina Hillson, Edward Buchanan, and Mafudia Suaray

Abbreviations

BV	Bacterial vaginosis
CDC	The centers for disease control and prevention
CMT	Cervical motion tenderness
CRP	C-reactive protein
CT	Computed tomography
ESR	Erythrocyte sedimentation rate
IUD	Intrauterine device
MRI	Magnetic resonance imaging
OCs	Oral contraceptives
PEACH	The pelvic inflammatory disease evaluation and clinical health randomized trial
PID	Pelvic inflammatory disease
STD	Sexually transmitted disease
STI	Sexually transmitted infection
TOA	Tubo-ovarian abscess
US	Ultrasonography
WBC	White blood cell count

J.H. Barash, MD (✉)
Department of Family and Community Medicine, Thomas Jefferson University Hospital, Philadelphia, PA, USA
e-mail: joshua.barash@jefferson.edu

C. Hillson, MD • E. Buchanan, MD • M. Suaray, MD
Department of Family and Community Medicine, Thomas Jefferson University, Philadelphia, PA, USA

N.S. Skolnik et al. (eds.), *Sexually Transmitted Diseases: A Practical Guide for Primary Care*, Current Clinical Practice, DOI 10.1007/978-1-62703-499-9_5,
© Springer Science+Business Media New York 2013

Introduction

Pelvic inflammatory disease (PID) is defined as an infection of the upper genital tract (uterus, fallopian tubes, and adjacent pelvic structures) that most commonly occurs among young, sexually active women. It is most often caused by the genital pathogens *Chlamydia trachomatis* and *Neisseria gonorrhoeae* and can be difficult to diagnose. An estimated 10–20 % of women with chlamydia or gonorrhea may develop PID if they do not receive adequate treatment. Among women with PID, tubal scarring can cause infertility in 20 % of women, ectopic pregnancy in 9 %, and chronic pelvic pain in 18 % [1, 2].

Epidemiology

Because PID is not a reportable disease, it is difficult to accurately quantify the number of women affected by PID on an annual basis. The Centers for Disease Control and Prevention (CDC), through an analysis of outpatient and hospital discharge codes, estimates that more than 750,000 women experience an episode of acute PID each year. Overall, this represents a decreasing trend over the past 10 years. However, since a large proportion of PID cases are unrecognized or subclinical, it is unclear whether this represents a true decrease in incidence. Racial disparities may also exist. Disease rates have been found to be 2–3 times higher among African-American women than among Caucasian women, which are consistent with the marked racial disparities observed for both chlamydia and gonorrhea. However, given the subjective methods by which PID is diagnosed, racial disparity data may be inaccurate [3].

Risk Factors

Young women with multiple partners are at greatest risk of developing PID. This may be partly due to an immature cervix that predisposes them to the common organisms that are responsible for causing PID. Nonuse of a barrier method also increases one's risk of developing PID; condoms with nonoxynol-9 provide increased protection [4]. A previous history of PID increases the risk for subsequent episodes [5]. In the past, it was thought that an intrauterine device (IUD) increased one's risk of developing PID. Modern IUDs cause little, if any, increased risk. Women who have an IUD inserted may have a slightly increased risk of PID near the time of insertion. However, this risk is greatly reduced if a woman is tested and, if necessary, treated for STDs before the IUD is inserted. Combined oral contraceptives (OCs) have shown a protective effect in some studies but not in others [6]. Current research suggests that OCs do not decrease the *incidence* of developing PID

Table 5.1 Risk factors for pelvic inflammatory disease

Known factors	Young age
	Multiple sexual partners
	Prior history of PID
	Sexually transmitted infection (gonorrhea, chlamydia)
	Lack of barrier contraceptive usage
Proposed factors (causative relationship not established)	Low socioeconomic status
	African-American
	Douching
	Urban living
	High frequency of sexual intercourse
	Coitus during menstruation
	Cigarette smoking
	Substance abuse

but do reduce the *severity* of PID [7]. Table 5.1 lists known risk factors for PID, as well as those that have been proposed but for which a causative relationship has not been established.

Microbiology

PID is a polymicrobial infection involving sexually transmitted organisms as well as aerobic and anaerobic vaginal microbes. The major initiating organisms usually implicated are *Neisseria gonorrhoeae* (*N. Gonorrhoeae*) and *Chlamydia Trachomatis* (*C. Trachomatis*); together they account for about 50 % of PID cases [8]. In at least one-third of PID cases, mixed infection involving both aerobic and anaerobic organisms is seen. Mycoplasma species, especially *M. genitalium*, are increasingly being recognized as a cause of non-chlamydial, nongonococcal PID [9]. Bacterial Vaginosis (BV)-associated organisms, such as *Gardnerella Vaginalis* and Bacteroides, have also been implicated in PID although BV alone has not been shown to be responsible [8, 10, 11]. In persons with BV, acquiring a gonococcal or chlamydial infection can result in a threefold increase in PID risk [12]. Other organisms frequently isolated in PID infections include *E. coli*, *Klebsiella* spp., Proteus, aerobic streptococci, and Peptostreptococcus [13–15].

Pathophysiology

The vaginal flora of most women consists of low numbers of potentially pathogenic organisms, among which are anaerobes, and species of Streptococci, Staphylococci, and Enterobacteriaceae [12]. The endocervical canal serves as a barrier to prevent organisms from entering the sterile upper genital tract. Cervical mucus has bacteriostatic properties. Hormonal changes affect the consistency of the cervical mucus plug. The cervical mucus gets thin during ovulation and the plug is lost at the onset of menses, granting pathogens access to the upper genital tract. Retrograde flow of menses is another mechanism that may explain the spread of the pathogens from the endometrium to the fallopian tubes. Protective elements of the endometrium are sloughed off during menses also predisposing to infection [16].

Infection by *N. gonorrhoeae*, *C. trachomatis*, and other organisms in the lower genital tract leads to a breakdown of cervical mucus which facilitates their spread via canalicular routes from the cervix to the structures of the upper genital tract. *N. gonorrhoeae* and *C. trachomatis* possess various membrane proteins that facilitate adherence to host epithelial cells and invasion of cells. They have also adapted mechanisms to evade and disrupt host defense mechanisms. *N. gonorrhoeae* possesses pili and other outer membrane structures that facilitate its attachment to mucosal cell linings, penetration, and destruction of epithelial cells. It destroys ciliary motility and causes distortion, distention, and subsequent obstruction of fallopian tubes. *C. trachomatis* possesses surface structures such as heat shock proteins and lipopolysaccharides that trigger a cytokine release and induce an inflammatory response which then leads to destruction of the mucosal cells lining the fallopian tubes [16, 17]. *M. genitalium* has also been shown to cause changes in ciliated fallopian tube cells that lead to salpingitis [9].

Diagnosis

As our understanding of the etiology and disease process involved in PID has improved, there has been a shift in the criteria used to diagnose PID. The traditional criteria outlined multiple decades ago required the presence of fever or leukocytosis, abdominal pain, cervical motion tenderness (CMT), and adnexal tenderness. Recent research has shown that only approximately 20 % of women with laparoscopically proven PID actually have this constellation of symptoms [15]. Because of the difficulty of diagnosis and the potential for damage to the reproductive health of women even by apparently mild or subclinical PID, the Center for Disease Control in 2010 altered their guidelines and recommended that healthcare providers maintain a low threshold for the diagnosis of PID [10, 18].

In the 2010 CDC guidelines (see Table 5.2), the criteria used to define PID was broadened to include sexually active young women (25 years old or younger) and other women at risk of sexually transmitted infections, with pelvic or abdominal pain (if no cause for the illness other than PID can be identified) and if either CMT, uterine tenderness or adnexal tenderness is present [10, 18]. The above approach is sufficient to assure that women with PID will be treated appropriately with antibiotics, but the criteria is not sensitive and up to a third of these women will not have acute PID [6, 19]. The specificity of the diagnosis can be increased if there is laboratory documentation of cervical infection with *N. gonorrhoeae* or *C. trachomatis* or

Table 5.2 CDC 2010 clinical diagnostic criteria for PID

PID is empirically treated in sexually active women experiencing pelvic or lower abdominal pain, if no other cause is identified and one of the following minimum criteria is present:
- Cervical motion tenderness
- Uterine tenderness
- Adnexal tenderness

The following criteria can improve the specificity of the diagnosis:
- Oral temperature > 101 °F (>38.3 °C)
- Abnormal cervical or vaginal mucopurulent discharge[a]
- Abundant numbers of white blood cells on saline microscopy of vaginal fluid[a]
- Elevated erythrocyte sedimentation rate
- Elevated C-reactive protein level
- Laboratory documentation of cervical infection with gonorrhea or chlamydia

The following test results are the most specific criteria for diagnosing PID:
- Endometrial biopsy with histopathologic evidence of endometritis
- Transvaginal sonography or magnetic resonance imaging techniques showing thickened, fluid-filled tubes with or without free pelvic fluid or tubo-ovarian complex, or Doppler studies suggesting pelvic infection (e.g., tubal hyperemia)
- Laparoscopic abnormalities consistent with PID

[a]Most women with PID have either mucopurulent discharge or evidence of WBCs on microscopy of vaginal fluid. If neither of these findings is present, PID is unlikely since this reliably excludes (negative predictive value 94.5 %) upper genital tract infection [10, 18]

Chart Source: Adapted from Centers for Disease Control and Prevention MMWR 2010;59 (No. RR-12):63–67 [35]. Accessed at http://www.cdc.gov/mmwr/preview/mmwrhtml/rr5912a1.htm 2/19/2013

signs of lower genital tract inflammation (predominance of leukocytes in vaginal secretions, cervical exudates, or cervical friability). If the cervix is normal and no white blood cells are noted during microscopy of the vaginal secretions, an alternative diagnosis should be investigated since this reliably excludes (negative predictive value 94.5 %) upper genital tract infection [10, 18].

History and Physical Examination

The diagnosis is based primarily on clinical evaluation and is challenging because symptoms can range from absent to subtle to severe [20]. Symptoms to screen for include abdominal pain, dyspareunia, fever, back pain, nausea, and vomiting, as well as symptoms of lower genital tract infection such as abnormal vaginal discharge and abnormal vaginal bleeding. Women with longer-standing disease can develop Fitz-Hugh Curtis Syndrome (see "Sequealae" section) and may complain of right upper quadrant pain due to perihepatitis. A key part in taking the history is screening for the risk factors for PID discussed above and in Table 5.1.

When conducting the physical exam, the examiner should take a full set of vital signs looking for fever and vital sign instability, as well as perform a thorough abdominal and pelvic examination. On abdominal exam one should evaluate for tenderness, the presence of a mass, rebound, guarding, or peritoneal signs. One should also carefully examine the right upper quadrant to assess for Fitz-Hugh-Curtis Syndrome. A bimanual pelvic exam must be performed to evaluate for CMT, uterine tenderness, or adnexal tenderness. The lower genital tract also needs to be assessed for signs of inflammation; thus a speculum exam is performed and the cervical canal examined for the presence of abnormal discharge and friability.

Laboratory

Microscopy of the vaginal secretions should be performed to evaluate for leukorrhea (more than 1 leukocyte per epithelial cell), bacterial vaginosis (vaginal pH, clue cells, and whiff test), and trichomonas vaginitis. Testing for *Neisseria gonorrhoeae* and *Chlamydia trachomatis* should also be performed.

Other laboratory tests are not part of routine diagnosis but can be helpful in supporting the diagnosis and monitoring response to treatment. Specifically, an elevated white blood cell count (WBC), erythrocyte sedimentation rate (ESR), or C-reactive protein (CRP) level can be helpful [10, 18]. WBC counts are beneficial when elevated, yet only 60 % of patients with PID will present with an elevated serum WBC count. An elevated ESR (>15 mm/h) is present in 75 % of women with PID but it is nonspecific. CRP levels >10 mg/dL have a relatively good sensitivity (93 %) and specificity (83 %) in the diagnosis of PID and CRP levels decrease to normal more rapidly than ESR following effective antibiotic therapy and may be beneficial as a monitoring tool [10, 18]. Research is also being done to evaluate the role of CA-125 in diagnosing PID. Studies show that elevated CA-125 levels confirm the diagnosis of peritoneal involvement in patients with a clinical diagnosis of PID and the level correlates with the extent of inflammatory peritoneal involvement. The predictive value of an elevated serum CA-125 level to indicate the presence of salpingitis is 97 %. However, the predictive value of a normal CA-125 level indicating normal observations at laparoscopy is only 47 % [10, 18].

Imaging

Routine imaging is not indicated to make the diagnosis of PID, but can play a role if one needs to rule out a competing diagnosis (e.g., an ultrasound to rule out ovarian cyst, a CT to rule out appendicitis), if a patient fails to respond to treatment, or if there is concern for complications arising from PID such as a tubo-ovarian abscess (TOA). Ultrasonography (US) is the first-line imaging technique for detecting PID because it is noninvasive, relatively inexpensive, and widely available. The transvaginal approach is preferred and the sensitivity is increased when performed with doppler flow. It has a sensitivity, specificity, and accuracy all around 80 % [21].

The specific finding of thickened fluid-filled tubes by ultrasonogaphy supports the diagnosis of upper genital tract inflammation.

If ultrasound is not adequate, the next step in imaging is magnetic resonance imaging (MRI). While MRI is significantly more expensive, it is more specific and accurate than ultrasound, with a sensitivity of 95 %, a specificity of 89 %, and an accuracy of 93 % [21]. Computed tomography (CT) should be reserved to assess the extent of the infection within the abdominal cavity and for interventional therapy to drain pelvic abscesses [15].

Surgery

Laparoscopy has been shown to add considerable accuracy to the clinical methods of diagnosing acute salpingitis. The procedure does not aggravate the inflammatory process. The minimum laparoscopic criteria for visual diagnosis of acute salpingitis include pronounced hyperemia of the tubal surface, edema of the tubal wall, and, thirdly, a sticky exudate on the tubal surface and from the fimbriated ends when patent [10, 18]. However, this technique can fail to isolate endometritis. Therefore, if laparoscopy fails to make a diagnosis, an endometrial biopsy may be indicated to rule out endometritis. Demonstration of endometrial inflammation (presence of neutrophils and plasma cells) on biopsy has both good sensitivity (70–80 %) and specificity (67–89 %) [15].

Treatment and Management

PID is treated on an empiric basis because a definitive diagnosis is rare and confirmatory tests are rarely known at diagnosis. Treatment should not be delayed because prevention of long-term sequelae due to this ascending infection is dependent on early administration of appropriate antibiotics [10, 18]. The first step in treatment is determining if either inpatient or outpatient management is necessary. Mild-to-moderate disease can be treated with similar efficacy with either inpatient or outpatient therapy. This recommendation is based on the pelvic inflammatory disease evaluation and clinical health randomized trial (PEACH) that showed that women with mild-to-moderate PID had similar short-term cure rates (both >98 %) when treated in either an inpatient (parenteral antibiotics) or outpatient setting (oral antibiotics). There was also no difference in the long-term outcomes of fertility and ectopic pregnancies between the two groups [6].

Hospitalization is necessary when any of the following criteria are met: a surgical emergency (e.g., appendicitis) cannot be excluded; the patient is pregnant; the patient does not respond clinically to oral antimicrobial therapy; the patient is unable to follow or tolerate an outpatient oral regimen; the patient has severe illness, nausea and vomiting, or high fever; or the patient has a TOA [10, 18]. There is no evidence to

Table 5.3 CDC treatment recommendations for PID

Parenteral treatment

Recommended regimen A
- Cefotetan 2 g IV every 12 h ORCefoxitin 2 g IV every 6 h
- PLUS Doxycycline 100 mg orally or IV every 12 h

Recommended regimen B
- Clindamycin 900 mg IV every 8 h PLUS
- Gentamicin loading dose IV or IM (2 mg/kg body weight) followed by a maintenance dose (1.5 mg/kg body weight) every 8 h. A single daily dosing (3–5 mg/kg) can be substituted

Alternative parenteral regimen
- Ampicillin/Sulbactam 3 g IV every 6 h
- PLUSDoxycycline 100 mg orally or IV every 12 h

Oral treatment

Recommended regimen A
- Ceftriaxone 250 mg IM in a single dose
- PLUS Doxycycline 100 mg orally twice a day for 14 days
- WITH OR WITHOUT Metronidazole 500 mg orally twice a day for 14 days

Recommended regimen B
- Cefoxitin 2 g IM in a single dose and Probenecid 1 g orally administered concomitantly as a single dose
- PLUS Doxycycline 100 mg orally twice a day for 14 days
- WITH OR WITHOUT Metronidazole 500 mg orally twice a day for 14 days

Alternative regimen
- Other parenteral third generation cephalosporins (e.g., ceftizoxime or cefotaxime) in a single dose
- PLUS Doxycycline 100 mg orally twice a day for 14 days
- WITH OR WITHOUT Metronidazole 500 mg orally twice a day for 14 day

Source: Adapted from: Centers for Disease Control and Prevention. Sexually Transmitted Diseases Treatment Guidelines, 2010. MMWR 2010;59(No. RR- 12):63–67 [35]. Accessed at http://www.cdc.gov/mmwr/preview/mmwrhtml/rr5912a1.htm 2/19/2013

suggest that adolescents benefit from hospitalization for treatment of PID. The decision to hospitalize adolescents with acute PID should be based on the same criteria used for older women [10, 18]. Women with HIV can also be treated according to the same criteria but clinicians must be aware that they are at increased risk for developing a tubo-ovarian abscess. Studies have also demonstrated more prolonged hospitalization among HIV seropositive women with acute salpingitis [21, 22].

The next step in management is choosing the appropriate antibiotic regimen (see Table 5.3). A broad-spectrum antibiotic regimen that targets a polymicrobial infection and addresses current resistance patterns is essential. Guidelines are frequently updated to reflect emerging resistance patterns and should be reviewed. All regimens used to treat PID should be effective against *N. gonorrhoeae* and *C. trachomatis*, even if cultures are negative, because negative endocervical screening for these organisms does not rule out upper reproductive tract infection. Current regimens also recommend covering anaerobes because anaerobic bacteria have been isolated from the upper reproductive tract of women who have PID, and data from in vitro studies have revealed that some anaerobes (e.g., *Bacteroides fragilis*) can cause tubal and epithelial destruction. BV is also present in many women who have PID [10, 18]. Until treatment regimens that do not adequately cover these microbes have been demonstrated to prevent long-term sequelae (e.g., infertility and ectopic pregnancy) as successfully as the regimens that are effective against these microbes, the use of regimens with anaerobic activity should be considered.

When parenteral therapy is indicated the preferred regimen is a cephalosporin (either Cefotetan or Cefoxitin) given in addition to doxycycline. Doxycycline has equal efficacy when administered orally or parenterally, and given the pain associated with infusion, the preferred route is oral. Preference is given to Cefotetan and Cefoxitin over other cephalosporins because they are more active against anaerobes than the other second- and third-generation cephalosporins. One can transition to oral therapy within 24–48 h of clinical improvement and then a complete 14-day course of oral antibiotics should be given [10, 18]. When a TOA is present, at least 24 h of inpatient observation is recommended. Clindamycin or metronidazole with doxycycline can then be used for continued therapy rather than doxycycline alone because this regimen provides more effective anaerobic coverage [10, 18]. Multiple alternative regimens exist for parenteral administration and are outlined in Table 5.3.

The current recommended outpatient regimen includes ceftriaxone given intramuscularly in one dose with doxycycline, with or without metronidazole. Alternative regimens are outlined in Table 5.3 and use other cephalosporins such as Cefoxitin which has improved anaerobe coverage over Ceftriaxone, but poorer coverage against *N. gonorrhea*. The metronidazole is added for additional anaerobic coverage and for treating bacterial vaginosis.

Sequelae

PID can cause complications that may increase a woman's risk for significant morbidity. During the infectious period, the development of Fitz-Hugh-Curtis syndrome or TOA may complicate diagnosis and treatment alternatives.

Fitz-Hugh-Curtis Syndrome

Women with PID are at risk for hematogenous or peritoneal spread of infection to the abdominal right upper quadrant resulting in perihepatitis. This manifests as right upper quadrant pain and tenderness with possible referred pain to the shoulder in 5 % of patients. Liver enzyme abnormalities may be detected and perihepatic inflammation may be noted on CT scan. Abnormal findings resolve with treatment of PID although the classic fiddle string appearance of hepatic adhesions to the anterior abdominal wall may be observed by laparoscopy years after the episode.

Tubo-Ovarian Abscess

Tubo-ovarian abscesses are inflammatory masses involving the fallopian tube, ovary, and surrounding structures. The true incidence of TOA is unknown although studies have shown 35 % of women hospitalized with PID have evidence of TOA by ultrasound [23–25].

Like PID, tubo-ovarian abscesses are polymicrobial in nature with *E. coli*, *B. fragilis*, and other Bacteroides species most commonly cultured from abscess fluid. Although *N. gonorrhea* has only rarely and *C. trachomatis* has never been isolated from TOA contents, the presence of these organisms in the endocervix appears to increase the risk of abscess formation [25].

The presence of a TOA may go undiagnosed since its symptoms are often attributed to the broader condition of PID and physical exam has low sensitivity in detecting pelvic masses. The use of ultrasound has improved detection rates with sensitivity and specificity of 93 % and 98.6 % respectively based on retrospective studies. Only one prospective study of the diagnostic use of ultrasound appears in the literature which reports a more modest 56 % sensitivity and 86 % specificity [26]. Further evaluation of imaging modalities including ultrasound, CT scan, and MRI are warranted.

Treatment of TOA begins with broad-spectrum, parenteral antibiotics as recommended by the CDC for treatment of PID (see Table 5.3). Metronidazole or clindamycin are especially effective given their anaerobic coverage and ability to penetrate an abscess. Improvement should be assessed clinically. For patients without improvement, ultrasound or CT guided drainage can be performed for abscesses in accessible locations. Success rates of 93.4 % have been reported with this technique [27, 28]. Finally, surgical irrigation and drainage, unilateral salpingo-oophorectomy, hysterectomy with bilateral salpingo-oophorectomy may be warranted in a patient not responding to more conservative measures. These procedures should be individualized to each case with consideration of severity of disease and desire for future fertility.

Other Complications

Long-term sequelae of PID include infertility, ectopic pregnancy, and chronic pelvic pain all of which result from inflammatory damage to pelvic organs.

Infertility is a consequence of fallopian tube damage such as fimbrial clubbing, cilial dysfunction along the endosalpinx, and complete obstruction of the tube. After a single episode of PID, infertility rates of 11–18 % have been observed. The incidence of infertility is directly related to the severity of PID as well as the number of lifetime episodes [2, 29, 30]. Subacute chlamydial infections play an insidious role in tubal damage as evidenced by the similar extent of damage from both acute and subacute infections [31]. Tubal damage also increases the risk of ectopic pregnancy in women with a history of PID who are able to conceive. After one episode of PID, the odds ratio for an ectopic in subsequent pregnancy is 3.0 [29]. Likewise, women with a history of PID have a relative risk of 4.5 for developing chronic pelvic pain over controls [32].

Screening and Prevention

Primary prevention of PID is accomplished using similar strategies to prevent other STDs. The surest way to avoid transmission of STDs is to abstain from sexual intercourse, or to be in a monogamous relationship with a partner who has been tested and is known to be uninfected. For sexually active individuals, one of the most important means of prevention is through condom use [33]. Limiting the number of sexual partners is also effective.

Secondary prevention involves screening and treating sexually active women for *N. gonorrhoeae* and *C. trachomatis*, thus preventing lower genital tract infections from ascending. In doing so, the risk for developing PID is reduced [34]. The CDC recommends yearly chlamydia testing of all sexually active women younger than 25 years, and in those 25 years and older with risk factors. More frequent screening may be indicated for some women in high-risk groups [35].

Finally, there is emerging research to suggest that education and brief behavioral intervention may be effective in decreasing the recurrence of PID [36].

References

1. Weström L. Incidence, prevalence, and trends of acute pelvic inflammatory disease and its consequences in industrialized countries. Obstet Gynecol. 1980;138(7 Pt 2):880.
2. Haggerty CL, Gottlieb SL, Taylor BD, Low N, Xu F, Ness RB. Risk of sequelae after Chlamydia trachomatis genital infection in women. J Infect Dis. 2010;201 Suppl 2:S134–55.
3. Sutton MY, Sternberg M, Zaidi A, St Louis ME, Markowitz LE. Trends in pelvic inflammatory disease hospital discharges and ambulatory visits, United States, 1985–2001. Sex Transm Dis. 2005;32(12):778.
4. Niruthisard S, Chutivongse S, Roddy R. Use of nonoxynol-9 and reduction in rate of gonococcal and chlamydial cervical infections. Lancet. 1992;339(8806):1371–5.
5. Flesh G, Weiner J, Corlett Jr R, Boice C, Mishell Jr D, Wolf R. The intrauterine contraceptive device and acute salpingitis: a multifactor analysis. Obstet Gynecol. 1979;135(3):402.
6. Ness RB, Soper DE, Holley RL, Peipert J, Randall H, Sweet RL, et al. Hormonal and barrier contraception and risk of upper genital tract disease in the PID Evaluation and Clinical Health (PEACH) study. Obstet Gynecol. 2001;185(1):121–7.
7. Wolner-Hanssen P, Svensson L, et al. Laparoscopic findings and contraceptive use in women with signs and symptoms suggestive of acute salpingitis. Obstet Gynecol. 1985;66(2):233.
8. McMCormack W. Current concepts: pelvic inflammatory disease. N Engl J Med. 1994; 330(2):115.
9. Haggerty CL, Taylor BD. Mycoplasma genitalium: an emerging cause of pelvic inflammatory disease. Infect Dis Obstet Gynecol. 2011;2011:959816.

10. Soper DE. Pelvic inflammatory disease. Obstet Gynecol. 2010;116(2 Part 1):419.
11. Soper D, Brockwell N, Dalton H, Johnson D. Observations concerning the microbial etiology of acute salpingitis. Am J Obstet Gynecol. 1994;170(4):1008.
12. Ness RB, Hillier SL, Kip KE, Soper DE, Stamm CA, McGregor JA, et al. Bacterial vaginosis and risk of pelvic inflammatory disease. Obstet Gynecol. 2004;104(4):761–9.
13. Lurie SS. Uterine cervical non-gonococcal and non-chlamydial bacterial flora and its antibiotic sensitivity in women with pelvic inflammatory disease: did it vary over 20 years? Isr Med Assoc J. 2010;12(12):747–50.
14. Creatsas GK, Pavlatos MP, Koumantakis E. Bacteriologic aspects of pelvic inflammatory disease in gynecologic patients. Gynecol Obstet Invest. 1982;13(1):1–8.
15. Sweet RL. Pelvic inflammatory disease: current concepts of diagnosis and management. Curr Infect Dis Rep. 2012;14:194–203.
16. Likis F. Upper genital tract infections in women. In: Nelson A, Wodward J, editors. Sexually transmitted diseases: a practical guide for primary care. Totowa, NJ: Humana Press; 2007. p. 183–203.
17. Scheuerpflug I, Rudel T, Ryll R, Pandit J, Meyer T. Roles of PilC and PilE proteins in pilus-mediated adherence of Neisseria gonorrhoeae and Neisseria meningitidis to human erythrocytes and endothelial and epithelial cells. Infect Immun. 1999;67(2):834–43.
18. Workowski KA, Berman S. Sexually transmitted diseases treatment guidelines, 2010. MMWR Recomm Rep. 2010;59(RR-12):1–110.
19. Jaiyeoba O, Soper DE. A practical approach to the diagnosis of pelvic inflammatory disease. Infect Dis Obstet Gynecol. 2011;2011:753037.
20. Crossman S. The challenge of pelvic inflammatory disease. Am Fam Physician. 2006;73(5):859–64.
21. Li W, Zhang Y, Cui Y, Zhang P, Wu X. Pelvic inflammatory disease: evaluation of diagnostic accuracy with conventional MR with added diffusion-weighted imaging. Abdom Imaging. 2013;38(1):193–200.
22. Stroger J. Gynecologic issues in the HIV infected woman. Infect Dis Clin North Am. 2008;22:709–39.
23. Landers D, Sweet R. Current trends in the diagnosis and treatment of tuboovarian abscess. Obstet Gynecol. 1985;151(8):1098.
24. McNeeley S, Hendrix SL, Mazzoni MM, Kmak DC, Ransom SB. Medically sound, cost-effective treatment for pelvic inflammatory disease and tuboovarian abscess. Obstet Gynecol. 1998;178(6):1272–8.
25. Rosen M, Breitkopf D, Waud K. Tubo-ovarian abscess management options for women who desire fertility. Obstet Gynecol Surv. 2009;64(10):681.
26. Lee DC, Swaminathan AK. Sensitivity of ultrasound for the diagnosis of tubo-ovarian abscess: a case report and literature review. J Emerg Med. 2011;40(2):170–5.
27. Gjelland K, Ekerhovd E, Granberg S. Transvaginal ultrasound-guided aspiration for treatment of tubo-ovarian abscess: a study of 302 cases. Obstet Gynecol. 2005;193(4):1323–30.
28. Lareau SM, Beigi RH. Pelvic inflammatory disease and tubo-ovarian abscess. Infect Dis Clin North Am. 2008;22(4):693–708.
29. Ness RB, Soper DE, Holley RL, Peipert J, Randall H, Sweet RL, et al. Effectiveness of inpatient and outpatient treatment strategies for women with pelvic inflammatory disease: results from the Pelvic Inflammatory Disease Evaluation and Clinical Health (PEACH) Randomized Trial. Obstet Gynecol. 2002;186(5):929–37.
30. Weström L, Joesoef R, Reynolds G, Hagdu A, Thompson SE. Pelvic inflammatory disease and fertility. A cohort study of 1,844 women with laparoscopically verified disease and 657 control women with normal laparoscopic results. Sex Transm Dis. 1992;19(4):185.
31. Patton DL, Moore DE, et al. A comparison of the fallopian tube's response to overt and silent salpingitis. Obstet Gynecol. 1989;73(4):622.
32. Buchan H, Vessey M, Goldacre M, Fairweather J. Morbidity following pelvic inflammatory disease. BJOG. 1993;100(6):558–62.

33. Hook III EW. An ounce of prevention. Ann Intern Med. 2005;143(10):751–2.
34. Scholes D, Stergachis A, Heidrich FE, Andrilla H, Holmes KK, Stamm WE. Prevention of pelvic inflammatory disease by screening for cervical chlamydial infection. N Engl J Med. 1996;334(21):1362–6.
35. Workowski KA, Berman S. Sexually transmitted diseases treatment guidelines, 2010. MMWR Recomm Rep 2010;59(RR-12):1–110. http://www.cdc.gov/mmwr/preview/mmwrhtml/rr5912a1.htm Accessed 19 Feb 2013.
36. Trent M, Chung S, Burke M, Walker A, Ellen JM. Results of a randomized controlled trial of a brief behavioral intervention for pelvic inflammatory disease in adolescents. J Pediatr Adolesc Gynecol. 2010;23(2):96–101.

Chapter 6
Viral Hepatitis

Justin A. Reynolds and Jeremy Herman

Abbreviations

ALT	Alanine aminotransferase
CDC	Centers for Disease Control and Prevention
dL	Deciliter
DNA	Deoxyribonucleic acid
EIA	Enzyme immunoassay
FDA	Food and Drug Administration
HAV	Hepatitis A virus
HBc	Hepatitis B core antigen
HBeAg	Hepatitis B e antigen
HBIG	Hepatitis B immunoglobulin
HBsAg	Hepatitis B surface antigen
HBV	Hepatitis B virus
HCC	Hepatocellular carcinoma
HCV	Hepatitis C virus
HIV	Human immunodeficiency virus
IG	Pooled immunoglobulin
IgG	Immunoglobulin G
IgM	Immunoglobulin M
IM	Intramuscular

J.A. Reynolds, MD (✉)
Division of Digestive Diseases, Department of Medicine,
David Geffen School of Medicine at UCLA, 11301 Wilshire BLVD,
BLDG 115, Room 215, Los Angeles, CA 90073, USA
e-mail: justinaaronreynolds@gmail.com

J. Herman, MD
Department of Medicine, Division of Gastroenterology, Cedars Sinai Medical Center,
8536 Wilshire Boulevard, #202, Beverly Hills, CA, USA

N.S. Skolnik et al. (eds.), *Sexually Transmitted Diseases: A Practical Guide for Primary Care*, Current Clinical Practice, DOI 10.1007/978-1-62703-499-9_6,
© Springer Science+Business Media New York 2013

IU	International units
mg	Milligram
MSM	Men who have sex with men
PCR	Polymerase chain reaction
peg-IFN	Pegylated-interferon
RIBA	Recombinant immunoblot assay
RNA	Ribonucleic acid
STI	Sexually transmitted infection
SVR	Sustained virologic response
US	United States

Hepatitis A

Epidemiology and Transmission

Hepatitis A virus (HAV) is the most common cause of acute infectious hepatitis world-wide. Although HAV is not typically considered a sexually transmitted infection (STI), sexual practices may contribute to its transmission and so HAV must always be considered in suspected cases of viral hepatitis. In the United States (US) the incidence of acute hepatitis A has declined substantially since vaccination was first instituted for high-risk individuals and children living in states with high rates of HAV [1]. Between 1995 and 2007, the incidence of acute HAV declined by 92 % from 12 cases per 100,000 to 1 case per 100,000. This decline was most pronounced in states where children were routinely vaccinated. By 2010, the nationwide incidence had fallen to 0.5 cases per 100,000 individuals, amounting to only 1,670 documented cases in total [2].

HAV is a single-stranded non-enveloped RNA virus from the *Picornaviridae* family, with an enterohepatic life cycle that enables fecal-oral transmission through contact with infectious sources [3]. Infection may occur via water, fomites, or under-cooked food sources, typically in combination with poor hygiene and sanitation. Travel to endemic countries (e.g., Mexico, Central/South America, Southeast Asia, etc.), person-to-person contact, community-wide outbreaks, exposure to daycare centers, and illegal drug use are the most common risk factors for acquisition [4]. Within the category of person-to-person contact, sexual transmission is an increasingly important contributor to HAV infection. Infection rates have steadily risen among men who have sex with men (MSM), but both heterosexual and homosexual behavior likely contribute to HAV transmission via apparent or gross fecal contamination [3, 5]. Some studies have also identified the number of sexual partners, frequent oral-anal contact, anal intercourse, or evidence of other STIs as risk factors [6].

Clinical Presentation and Treatment

HAV has an incubation period that ranges from 15 to 50 days before the onset of clinical symptoms. During this asymptomatic incubation period and into the symptomatic period of illness, HAV will be shed into the stool of the infected person, raising the risk of further transmission. In HAV-infected children under age 6, only 20 % will develop a clinical illness, whereas 70–80 % of adults will have overt symptoms [7]. Following the incubation period which averages 30 days, prodromal symptoms of malaise, fever, anorexia, right upper quadrant abdominal pain, nausea, and vomiting will develop. Within 1–2 weeks, the prodromal symptoms wane and the icteric phase begins with the development of dark urine, acholic (light-colored) stool, and progression to overt jaundice. This icteric phase typically peaks within 2 weeks. On physical exam, jaundice and hepatomegaly are the most common findings. Lab tests typically reveal markedly abnormal serum aminotransferases, frequently over 1,000 IU/dL, and a mixed hyperbilirubinemia commonly above 10 mg/dL that peaks after the aminotransferases begin to improve. Positive testing for anti-HAV immunoglobulin M (IgM) in a symptomatic patient indicates acute infection, and typically can be detected 5–10 days before the onset of symptoms and may persist for up to 6 months following infection. Previous exposure or immunization is reflected in testing of anti-HAV IgG.

HAV is most often a self-limited acute illness that does not cause chronic infection, although a relapsing hepatitis can occur in 5–20 % of patients [8]. These patients have a prolonged course of jaundice, viral shedding, and infectivity. Treatment for hepatitis A infection, in general, is supportive, although occasionally hospitalization is necessary because of dehydration or food intolerance. In less than 1 % of all cases, HAV can present with fulminant liver failure, characterized by progressive jaundice, prolonged prothrombin time, and encephalopathy. Viral genotypic variations may contribute to this [9, 10], but the development of fulminant hepatitis is likely due in part to a vigorous host immune response as well [11]. Patients 50 years of age and older, and those with other underlying liver disease (e.g., chronic hepatitis B or C, alcoholic liver disease) are at increased risk for fulminant liver failure [12]. In these patients, liver transplantation can be lifesaving.

Prevention and Prophylaxis

Public health practices like improved personal hygiene during food preparation, improved sanitation of water processing and sewage disposal, and reduced contact with infected individuals will all help diminish HAV transmission. In addition, certain individuals are recommended HAV vaccination based on guidelines put forth by the Centers for Disease Control and Prevention (CDC) Advisory Committee on Immunization Practices. Currently HAV vaccination is recommended for all MSM, as well as any individual with another risk factor for HAV acquisition [13]. Such risk factors include travel or work in countries with intermediate or high endemicity of HAV, daycare workers, users of intravenous drugs, etc.

Hepatitis A vaccines are prepared from formalin-inactivated, cell-culture-derived HAV, and have been available in the US since 1995 [14]. The vaccine is administered intramuscularly (IM) in a two-dose series at 0 and 6–12 months. By 1 month after the first dose, approximately 95 % of adults have protective antibody levels.

Combination vaccines incorporating hepatitis A and hepatitis B are also available as a three-dose series administered according to a 0-, 1-, and 6-month schedule. As HAV vaccination becomes more commonplace, anti-HAV seroprevalence increases which can lead to a "herd immunity" and diminish the likelihood of future outbreaks. This effect is mitigated, however, by travel to endemic areas, importation of fruits/vegetables from endemic regions, etc.

In nonimmune persons already exposed to HAV or in whom active vaccination will not provide timely protection, passive immunization via intramuscular administration of pooled human immunoglobulin (IG) is recommended. If administered before or within 2 weeks of exposure to HAV, IG is effective in preventing progression to clinical disease in >85 % of cases [14]. However, receiving IG will not confer long-term immunity, so HAV vaccination should be considered at the time of IG administration. These may be administered concomitantly at different anatomical sites; however, IG may decrease immunogenicity of other concomitantly administered attenuated live vaccines (e.g., measles, mumps, rubella). IG is also contraindicated in patients with selective IgA deficiency because of reports of anaphylaxis.

Hepatitis B

Epidemiology and Transmission

Over 300 million persons worldwide are carriers of Hepatitis B virus (HBV), with approximately 1.25 million HBV carriers in the US [15]. The worldwide prevalence of HBV carriers varies from 0.1 to 2.0 % in low prevalence areas (e.g., the US, Canada, Australia), 3–5 % in intermediate prevalence regions (e.g., Japan, Central/South America, Middle East), and 10–20 % in high prevalence areas (e.g., China, Southeast Asia, sub-Saharan Africa) [16]. With increased HBV vaccination of all children and at-risk adults, as well as perinatal HBV screening of all pregnant mothers, there was an 81 % decline in the incidence of acute hepatitis B cases between 1990 and 2006 in the US [17]. Despite this, in 2007 there were an estimated 43,000 new cases of HBV, the majority of which were in adult men ages 25–44. In these individuals, the most common risk factors were intravenous drug use and sexual contact (e.g., having sex with an HBV carrier, multiple sexual partners, MSM, etc.). Thus, despite the success of vaccination, the burden of disease remains high. This has tremendous implications as carriers of HBV are at increased risk of cirrhosis, hepatocellular carcinoma (HCC), and death from chronic liver disease.

HBV is a double-stranded DNA hepadnavirus with multiple genotypes that vary geographically. HBV is found at highest concentrations within the blood, but may also be found in bodily fluids like semen or vaginal secretions. The primary mode of transmission of HBV varies based on the geographical region. In high prevalence areas, perinatal infection (or vertical transmission) is most common. This may occur in utero, during childbirth, or after delivery. Routine Caesarean section has not been proven to diminish the risk of maternal–infant transmission and is not recommended. In moderate prevalence areas, horizontal transmission is most common and generally occurs through minor cuts or breaks in the skin or mucous membranes via the sharing of household items (e.g., razors, toothbrush, etc.).

In low prevalence areas like the US, sexual contact and intravenous drug use are the primary modes of transmission. Nearly 25 % of regular sexual contacts of HBV-infected persons will become HBV-positive [18]. Heterosexual contact is estimated to account for 39 % of new HBV infections, and MSM transmission is estimated to account for 24 % of new cases [17]. Intravenous drug use is estimated to account for 16 % of new cases, and the risk of acquiring HBV varies based upon length of drug abuse, sharing of equipment, frequency of drug use, etc. However, even brief drug use can expose a patient to significant risk, as the risk of transmission via percutaneous exposure (e.g., needle-stick injury, tattoo, intravenous drug use) is estimated as high as 30 % [19].

Clinical Presentation and Treatment

Infection with HBV can result in an acute and self-limited illness, fulminant hepatitis, or it may lead to a chronic carrier state. The incubation period of HBV ranges from 1 to 4 months during which time the patient is asymptomatic but may infect others. Prodromal symptoms may then develop, and are nonspecific and include malaise, anorexia, nausea, myalgias, and right upper quadrant abdominal pain. The icteric phase follows and typically lasts 1–3 weeks and is characterized by jaundice, light-colored stools, dark urine, and tender hepatomegaly. The convalescent stage is characterized by malaise and fatigue which can persist for weeks to months. Less than 1 % of acute infections will result in hepatic decompensation and fulminant liver failure. When this occurs, it is felt to be the result of overwhelming immune-mediated hepatocyte destruction. Many of these patients will have no evidence of active HBV replication despite worsening liver failure [20].

If infected with HBV as an infant, over 90 % will be clinically asymptomatic but go on to have chronic HBV. Children infected between ages 1 and 5 will progress to chronic HBV in 20–50 % of affected children. On the contrary, less than 5 % of persons infected with HBV during adulthood will progress on to chronic HBV [21]. Patients with chronic HBV can be completely asymptomatic and can have a normal physical exam and laboratory tests. However, they will frequently have asymptomatic elevations in serum alanine aminotransferase (ALT) that fluctuate over time. If their liver disease progresses, they may develop signs of hepatic decompensation such as jaundice, ascites, and encephalopathy. Chronic carriers of HBV can also develop HCC, even in the absence of cirrhosis. Occasionally the clue to diagnosing HBV is the development of an extrahepatic manifestation such as polyarteritis nodosa or membranoproliferative glomerulonephritis [22, 23]. These are thought to arise as a result of immune complex deposition in end-organs. Antiviral therapy directed at HBV may have a role in the treatment of these two entities [24, 25].

In all HBV carrier states, prolonged viral replication and immune clearance of HBV-infected hepatocytes can ultimately lead to progressive liver fibrosis [26]. Progression to cirrhosis is also more likely in patients co-infected with hepatitis C or human immunodeficiency virus (HIV) [27], or in those who have an elevated ALT or are positive for hepatitis B e antigen (HBeAg) [28–30]. HBV carriers can also develop severe flares of viremia and transaminemia during periods of immunosuppression (e.g., chemotherapy, bone marrow transplant, glucocorticoid use, etc.) that can lead to acute liver failure. This has also been documented to occur in HBV-infected patients who have previously seroconverted and apparently resolved their infection [31]. In these patients, the risk of reactivation appears to be highest as the immunosuppression resolves and the newly reconstituted immune system aggressively attacks HBV-infected hepatocytes. Initiation of antiviral therapy is urgent, but despite this, some patients will still ultimately require liver transplantation. In cases where HBV status is known and immunosuppression is anticipated, antiviral therapy should be strongly considered.

If HBV infection is suspected, the diagnosis can be confirmed through serological testing. In general, the presence of hepatitis B surface antigen (HBsAg) is the hallmark of HBV infection, and this appears in serum within weeks of exposure to HBV. During this time, IgM antibodies to hepatitis B core antigen (IgM-HBc) are also positive. As the acute infection resolves, HBsAg disappears and the only serologic marker of acute HBV is IgM-HBc. This period between the disappearance of HBsAg and the emergence of hepatitis B surface antibody (anti-HBs) is called the "window period." After anti-HBs appears in the serum, the patient is generally felt to have resolved their infection. In rare cases, HBsAg and anti-HBs coexist as the antibodies are unable to neutralize circulating virions. These patients should be regarded as chronic carriers of HBV [32]. Chronic HBV is reflected by HBsAg that remains detectable for at least 6 months after infection, indicating active viral replication. The presence of anti-HBc and anti-HBs are indicative of cleared, inactive infection. The presence of anti-HBs alone indicates prior immunization to HBV.

For acute HBV infections, treatment is supportive. Some individuals will require hospitalization because of the inability to tolerate oral intake, or concern over progression to fulminant liver disease. If the infection persists into the chronic phase, treatment options include the use of nucleoside reverse transcriptase inhibitors like tenofovir, entecavir, telbivudine, adefovir, or lamivudine. Interferon is also used in certain circumstances. However, many HBV carriers do not need active antiviral treatment, but rather close monitoring and HCC screening. These decisions are complex and outside the scope of this chapter, so these patients are best served by referral to a specialist with experience in hepatitis B treatment.

Prevention and Prophylaxis

The hepatitis B vaccine is safe, well-tolerated, and is recommended by the CDC for universal immunization of infants and previously unvaccinated children. Vaccination is also recommended for adults at risk for infection including MSM, intravenous drug users, healthcare workers, etc. Screening before vaccination is not cost-effective unless the population being assessed has a greater than 20 % risk of HBV infection [33].

Postexposure prophylaxis is recommended for all non-vaccinated individuals who come into contact with HBV-infected blood or bodily secretions. If the HBsAg status of the source is unknown or negative, HBV vaccination alone is recommended as postexposure prophylaxis. The first dose of HBV vaccine should be given within 12 hours, and the remainder of the vaccination series should be completed according to schedule. If the source is known to be HBsAg-positive, hepatitis B immunoglobulin (HBIG) should be administered concomitant with vaccination at a different anatomical site. In a person previously vaccinated against HBV who is then exposed to an HBV-infected source, the recommendations for postexposure prophylaxis vary depending on whether a postvaccination antibody response was assessed. If postvaccination antibody response (i.e., development of anti-HBs) is present, no prophylaxis is needed after exposure. If there was no antibody response to prior vaccination, the exposed person should receive HBIG and undergo repeat vaccination (alternatively they may receive two courses of HBIG, 1 month apart). If postvaccination antibody response is unknown, that individual should have anti-HBs titers checked. If positive, no treatment is necessary; if inadequate, HBIG and repeat vaccination should be given.

Hepatitis C

Epidemiology and Transmission

In the US, hepatitis C virus (HCV) is the most common cause of death from liver disease, and is the most common indication for liver transplantation [34]. The World Health Organization estimates that up to 170 million persons are infected worldwide. In the US, up to 3.2 million persons are thought to be infected, but some estimate that figure to be as high as 5 million persons due to underrepresentation in survey data [35]. The CDC estimates the incidence of new HCV infections has dropped from 230,000 per year in the 1980s to 19,000 per year in 2006 [17]. This decline likely represents greater awareness, preventative measures, and the ability to screen for HCV.

HCV is a single-stranded RNA virus from the *Flaviviridae* family, of which multiple genotypes exist. In the US, genotype 1 is the most prevalent (70 % of all HCV-infected persons), and also the most difficult to treat. Genotypes 2 and 3 follow in prevalence and constitute approximately 20–25 % of all HCV-infected persons. Exposures such as needle-stick injuries, conjunctival splashes, and sharing of household items (e.g., razors, toothbrushes, etc.) all confer a risk of HCV transmission. However, HCV is primarily transmitted through parenteral exposure to infected blood. Intravenous drug use is the most efficient means of HCV transmission and is a strong risk factor for acquisition of HCV. Prior studies have shown that persons with a history of intravenous drug use were nearly 50 times more likely to have HCV than matched controls [36]. The peak prevalence is noted in the "baby boom" generation of persons born between 1945 and 1964. Other persons considered high-risk for HCV include those with hemophilia, hemodialysis-dependence, history of transfusion pre-1990, and history of STIs.

There is no doubt that sexual transmission of HCV is possible, although the risk appears to be low. Prior retrospective studies have demonstrated a potential risk of transmission of 0.1 % annually between heterosexual, monogamous couples [37]. Another prospective study involving monogamous heterosexual pairs with a 10-year follow-up period demonstrated no definite intraspousal transmission of HCV [38]. Despite these studies, 15–20 % of HCV-infected persons report high-risk sexual behavior in the absence of other risk factors for HCV acquisition [39]. Sexual transmission may be more likely if the HCV-infected individual is also a carrier of HIV [40]. Vertical transmission from an HCV-infected pregnant mother to infant occurs in 5–6 % of cases [41]. This risk of vertical transmission is nearly twofold in mothers co-infected with HIV [42]. Viral infectivity is likely related, in part, to the degree of active viremia at the time of childbirth. Neither breastfeeding nor type of delivery appears to increase the risk of viral transmission.

Clinical Presentation and Treatment

HCV has an incubation period that averages 6–12 weeks in duration, and the majority of infections are subclinical and unnoticed by the infected individual. Fewer than 20 % of individuals will develop symptoms during their acute hepatitis [39]. If present, these symptoms are similar to those experienced in other forms of acute hepatitis: anorexia, malaise, nausea, vomiting, and jaundice. Fulminant liver failure from acute HCV infection is quite rare, but the risk may be higher in patients with underlying chronic HBV [43]. The majority of HCV-infected individuals develop a chronic hepatitis (60–80 %) characterized by active viremia and abnormal liver enzymes. Approximately 5–20 % of chronic HCV-infected persons will develop cirrhosis after 20 years of infection [44]. Many host-related factors and exposures are associated with progression to cirrhosis in HCV-infected persons. Strong associations include chronic alcohol intake, advanced age, male sex, and viral co-infection with HBV or HIV. Other likely associations include diabetes, obesity, and fatty liver disease. Extrahepatic manifestations of HCV are recognized and include mixed cryoglobulinemia, porphyria cutanea tarda, lichen planus, glomerulonephritis, autoimmune thyroiditis, and seronegative arthritis. Recognition of these entities should prompt an evaluation for HCV infection.

Screening for HCV should be done with anti-HCV enzyme immunoassay (EIA). The anti-HCV EIA typically becomes positive within 8 weeks of HCV infection, but in rare cases can take months to become positive. A positive anti-HCV has high positive predictive value, but must be confirmed with a secondary test and it cannot distinguish between acute and chronic infection. After obtaining a positive anti-HCV, an HCV RNA should then be drawn. If the HCV RNA is negative, a recombinant immunoblot assay (RIBA) should then be sent to distinguish a false-positive EIA from past or resolved HCV infection. A positive HCV RNA confirms the presence of HCV viremia and indicates infection, and if persistent beyond 6 months, chronic infection. Any patient with a risk factor for acquiring HCV should be screened. Risk factors for HCV include a history of at least one episode of injection drug use, blood transfusion prior to 1990, long-term hemodialysis, occupational exposure to HCV-positive blood, being a sexual partner to an HCV-infected person, etc.

Treatment of HCV is dependent upon numerous host factors, lack of contraindications, and the genotype of the HCV-infected person. The goal of treatment in these patients is to eradicate HCV RNA and achieve sustained virologic response (SVR), which is associated with decreased rates of HCC, liver-related mortality and complications, and need for liver transplantation. Achieving SVR is defined as a lack of HCV RNA 6 months after the end of treatment, and this implies a 99 % chance of being HCV RNA negative in the long-term [45]. If HCV is discovered during the acute hepatitis phase, there are some data to suggest that it is more likely to resolve spontaneously [46], even without antiviral therapy. In those with persistent viremia lasting 12 weeks beyond the onset of clinical symptoms, progression to chronic hepatitis is more likely and starting antiviral therapy may be of benefit. Several small studies examining the efficacy of interferon treatment for acute HCV have indicated promising results with SVR rates upwards of 90 % [47, 48]. Although heterogeneous and somewhat limited by small sample size or lack of randomization, these studies indicate a consistent benefit to early antiviral treatment in these patients. However, not enough data regarding ribavirin use, length of therapy, or type of interferon exist to present specific recommendations for antiviral treatment of acute HCV patients [49].

In patients with chronic HCV, pegylated-interferon (peg-IFN) and ribavirin were the standard of care treatment for all genotypes of HCV in recent years, although the dosing and duration varied depending on HCV genotype, prior treatment response, and the presence (or absence) of cirrhosis. Unfortunately, standard therapy with peg-IFN and ribavirin has been somewhat disappointing, particularly for genotype 1 chronic HCV patients with SVR rates averaging 45–55 % in treatment-naïve patients. SVR rates were even lower in patients with prior treatment failure, presence of cirrhosis, or specific genetic predispositions. In 2011, two new protease inhibitors, telaprevir and boceprevir, were FDA-approved for use in addition to peg-IFN and ribavirin in the treatment of HCV genotype 1, raising SVR rates in genotype 1 treatment-naïve patients to 70–80 % [50, 51]. These protease inhibitors also dramatically improved SVR rates among patients with relapsed HCV viremia, prior partial response, and null response to treatment. However, numerous drug–drug interactions exist, as well as severe side effects including cytopenias, rash, neurologic effects, renal injury, etc. Therefore, antiviral treatment in these patients is complex and should be deferred to an experienced provider.

Prevention

No vaccine is available to prevent the acquisition of HCV, and no forms of postexposure prophylaxis exist. Therefore, education of individuals at risk for transmitting or acquiring HCV remains the mainstay of primary prevention of HCV. Infected persons should not share household items that may be contaminated by blood such as razors, toothbrushes, nail clippers, etc. Persons who inject illicit drugs should cease, or at minimum use sterile syringes and equipment. Although the risk of acquiring HCV from an infected sexual partner is low, persons at risk for STIs should be counseled on general precautions to lower their risk of acquiring bloodborne STIs (e.g., HIV, HBV, HCV) by using barrier methods or sexual abstinence. Persons in a stable monogamous sexual relationship with an HCV-infected patient are not counseled to change their current sexual habits.

References

1. Daniels D, Grytdal S, Wasley A. Surveillance for acute viral hepatitis—United States, 2007. MMWR Surveill Summ. 2009;58(3):1–27.
2. Centers for Disease Control and Prevention. Viral hepatitis statistics & surveillance. Atlanta, GA: US Department of Health and Human Services, Centers for Disease Control and Prevention; 2004. Table 2.1 Reported cases of acute hepatitis A, by state—United States, 2006–2010. Available at: http://www.cdc.gov/hepatitis/Statistics/2010Surveillance/Table2.1.htm. Accessed 18 July 2012.
3. Cuthbert JA. Hepatitis A: old and new. Clin Microbiol Rev. 2001;14(1):38–58.
4. Klevens RM, Miller JT, Iqbal K, Thomas A, Rizzo EM, Hanson H, et al. The evolving epidemiology of hepatitis a in the United States: incidence and molecular epidemiology from population-based surveillance, 2005-2007. Arch Intern Med. 2010;170(20):1811–8.
5. Ross JDC, Ghanem M, Tariq A, Gilleran G, Winter AJ. Seroprevalence of hepatitis A immunity in male genitourinary medicine clinic attenders: a case control study of hetero-sexual and homosexual men. Sex Transm Infect. 2002;78:174–9.
6. Katz MH, Hsu L, Wong E, Liska S, Anderson L, Janssen RS. Seroprevalence of and risk factors for hepatitis A infection among young homosexual and bisexual men. J Infect Dis. 1997;175:1225–9.
7. Tong MJ, el-Farra NS, Grew MI. Clinical manifestations of hepatitis A: recent experience in a community teaching hospital. J Infect Dis. 1995;171 Suppl 1:S15–8.
8. Glikson M, Galun E, Oren R, Tur-Kaspa R, Shouval D. Relapsing hepatitis. A Review of 14 cases and literature survey. Medicine (Baltimore). 1992;71(1):14–23.
9. Fujiwara K, Yokosuka O, Ehata T, Saisho H, Saotome N, Suzuki K, et al. Association between severity of type A hepatitis and nucleotide variations in the 5′ non-translated region of hepatitis a virus RNA: strains from fulminant hepatitis have fewer nucleotide substitutions. Gut. 2002;51:82–8.
10. Hussain Z, Husain SA, Pasha ST, Anand R, Chand A, Polipalli SK, et al. Does mutation of hepatitis A virus exist in North India? Dig Dis Sci. 2008;53:506–10.
11. Rezende G, Roque-Afonso AM, Samuel D, Gigou M, Nicand E, Ferre V, et al. Viral and clinical factors associated with the fulminant course of hepatitis A infection. Hepatology. 2003;38:613–8.

12. Vento S, Garofano T, Renzini C, et al. Fulminant hepatitis associated with hepatitis A virus superinfection in patients with chronic hepatitis C. N Engl J Med. 1998;338:286–90.

13. Baker CJ, Bennett N, Bocchini Jr JA, Campos-Outcalt D, Coyne-Beasley T, Duchin J, et al. Recommended adult immunization schedule: United States, 2012. Ann Intern Med. 2012;156(3):211–7.

14. Workowski KA, Berman S. Sexually transmitted diseases treatment guidelines, 2010. MMWR Recomm Rep. 2010;59(RR-12):1–110.

15. Lee WM. Hepatitis B, virus infection. N Engl J Med. 1997;337:1733–45.

16. Maynard JE. Hepatitis B: global importance and need for control. Vaccine. 1990;8(Suppl):S18–20.

17. Wasley A, Grytdal S, Gallagher K, Centers for Disease Control and Prevention (CDC). Surveillance for acute viral hepatitis—United States, 2006. MMWR Surveill Summ. 2008;57(2):1.

18. Practice Committee of the American Society for Reproductive Medicine. Hepatitis and reproduction. Fertil Steril. 2004;82:1754–64.

19. Papaevangelou GJ, Roumeliotou-Karayannis AJ, Contoyannis PC. The risk of nosocomial hepatitis A and B virus infections from patients under care without isolation precaution. J Med Virol. 1981;7:143–8.

20. Wright TL, Mamish D, Combs C, Kim M, Donegan E, Ferrell L, et al. Hepatitis B virus and apparent fulminant non-A, non-B hepatitis. Lancet. 1992;339(8799):952–5.

21. Tassopoulos NC, Papaevangelou GJ, Sjogren MH, Roumeliotou-Karayannis A, Gerin JL, Purcell RH. Natural history of acute hepatitis B surface antigen-positive hepatitis in Greek adults. Gastroenterology. 1987;92(6):1844–50.

22. Guillevin L, Mahr A, Callard P, Godmer P, Pagnoux C, Leray E, et al. French Vasculitis Study Group. Hepatitis B virus-associated polyarteritis nodosa: clinical characteristics, outcome, and impact of treatment in 115 patients. Medicine (Baltimore). 2005;84(5):313–22.

23. Johnson RJ, Couser WG. Hepatitis B infection and renal disease: clinical, immunopathogenetic and therapeutic considerations. Kidney Int. 1990;37(2):663–76.

24. Janssen HL, van Zonneveld M, van Nunen AB, Niesters HG, Schalm SW, de Man RA. Polyarteritis nodosa associated with hepatitis B virus infection. The role of antiviral treatment and mutations in the hepatitis B virus genome. Eur J Gastroenterol Hepatol. 2004;16(8):801–7.

25. Zheng XY, Wei RB, Tang L, Li P, Zheng XD. Meta-analysis of combined therapy for adult hepatitis B virus-associated glomerulonephritis. World J Gastroenterol. 2012;18(8):821–32.

26. de Jongh FE, Janssen HL, de Man RA, Hop WC, Schalm SW, van Blankenstein M. Survival and prognostic indicators in hepatitis B surface antigen-positive cirrhosis of the liver. Gastroenterology. 1992;103(5):1630–5.

27. Colin JF, Cazals-Hatem D, Loriot MA, Martinot-Peignoux M, Pham BN, Auperin A, et al. Influence of human immunodeficiency virus infection on chronic hepatitis B in homosexual men. Hepatology. 1999;29(4):1306–10.

28. Yu MW, Hsu FC, Sheen IS, et al. Prospective study of hepatocellular carcinoma and liver cirrhosis in asymptomatic chronic hepatitis B virus carriers. Am J Epidemiol. 1997;145:1039–47.

29. Liaw YF, Tai DI, Chu CM, Chen TJ. The development of cirrhosis in patients with chronic type B hepatitis: a prospective study. Hepatology. 1988;8:493–6.

30. Realdi G, Fattovich G, Hadziyannis S, et al. Survival and prognostic factors in 366 patients with compensated cirrhosis type B: a multicenter study. The Investigators of the European Concerted Action on Viral Hepatitis (EUROHEP). J Hepatol. 1994;21:656–66.

31. Perrillo RP. Acute flares in chronic hepatitis B: the natural and unnatural history of an immunologically mediated liver disease. Gastroenterology. 2001;120(4):1009–22.

32. Tsang TK, Blei AT, O'Reilly DJ, Decker R. Clinical significance of concurrent hepatitis B surface antigen and antibody positivity. Dig Dis Sci. 1986;31(6):620–4.

33. Centers for Disease Control and Prevention. Hepatitis B. In: Atkinson W, Hamborsky J, Wolfe S, editors. Epidemiology and prevention of vaccine-preventable diseases. 8th ed. Washington, DC: Public Health Foundation; 2004. p. 191–212.

34. Kim WR. The burden of hepatitis C in the United States. Hepatology. 2002;36:S30–4.

35. Chak E, Talal AH, Sherman KE, Schiff ER, Saab S. Hepatitis C virus infection in USA: an estimate of true prevalence. Liver Int. 2011;31(8):1090–101.

36. Murphy EL, Bryzman SM, Glynn SA, Ameti DI, Thomson RA, Williams AE, et al. Risk factors for hepatitis C virus infection in United States blood donors. NHLBI Retrovirus Epidemiology Donor Study (REDS). Hepatology. 2000;31(3):756–62.

37. Dienstag JL. Sexual and perinatal transmission of hepatitis C. Hepatology. 1997;26(3 Suppl 1): 66S–70.

38. Vandelli C, Renzo F, Romanò L, Tisminetzky S, De Palma M, Stroffolini T, et al. Lack of evidence of sexual transmission of hepatitis C among monogamous couples: results of a 10-year prospective follow-up study. Am J Gastroenterol. 2004;99(5):855–9.

39. Centers for Disease Control and Prevention. Recommendations for prevention and control of hepatitis C virus (HCV) infection and HCV-related chronic disease. MMWR Recomm Rep. 1998;47:1–39.

40. Tohme RA, Holmberg SD. Is sexual contact a major mode of hepatitis C virus transmission? Hepatology. 2010;52(4):1497–505.

41. Ohto H, Terazawa S, Sasaki N, Sasaki N, Hino K, Ishiwata C, et al. Transmission of hepatitis C virus from mothers to infants. The Vertical Transmission of Hepatitis C Virus Collaborative Study Group. N Engl J Med. 1994;330(11):744–50.

42. Zanetti AR, Tanzi E, Paccagnini S, Principi N, Pizzocolo G, Caccamo ML, et al. Mother-to-infant transmission of hepatitis C virus. Lombardy Study Group on Vertical HCV Transmission. Lancet. 1995;345(8945):289–91.

43. Chu CM, Yeh CT, Liaw YF. Fulminant hepatic failure in acute hepatitis C: increased risk in chronic carriers of hepatitis B virus. Gut. 1999;45(4):613–7.

44. Seeff LB. Natural history of chronic hepatitis C. Hepatology. 2002;36:S35–46.

45. Swain MG, Lai MY, Shiffman ML, Cooksley WG, Zeuzem S, Dieterich DT, et al. A sustained virologic response is durable in patients with chronic hepatitis C treated with peginterferon alfa-2a and ribavirin. Gastroenterology. 2010;139(5):1593–601.

46. Gerlach JT, Diepolder HM, Zachoval R, Gruener NH, Jung MC, Ulsenheimer A, et al. Acute hepatitis C: high rate of both spontaneous and treatment-induced viral clearance. Gastroenterology. 2003;125(1):80–8.

47. Kamal SM, Moustafa KN, Chen J, Fehr J, Abdel Moneim A, Khalifa KE, et al. Duration of peginterferon therapy in acute hepatitis C: a randomized trial. Hepatology. 2006;43(5): 923–31.

48. Licata A, Di Bona D, Schepis F, Shahied L, Craxí A, Cammà C. When and how to treat acute hepatitis C? J Hepatol. 2003;39(6):1056–62.

49. Ghany MG, Strader DB, Thomas DL, Seeff LB, American Association for the Study of Liver Diseases. Diagnosis, management, and treatment of hepatitis C: an update. Hepatology. 2009;49(4):1335–74.

50. Jacobson IM, McHutchison JG, Dusheiko G, Di Bisceglie AM, Reddy KR, Bzowej NH, et al., ADVANCE Study Team. Telaprevir for previously untreated chronic hepatitis C virus infection. N Engl J Med. 2011;364(25):2405–16.

51. Poordad F, McCone J Jr, Bacon BR, Bruno S, Manns MP, Sulkowski MS, et al., SPRINT-2 Investigators. Boceprevir for untreated chronic HCV genotype 1 infection. N Engl J Med. 2011;364(13):1195–206.

Chapter 7
HIV: Identification, Diagnosis, and Prevention

Gunter Rieg

Introduction

In the summer of 1981, the Centers for Disease Control and Prevention (CDC) reported clusters of unusual infections (*Pneumocystis carinii* pneumonia, now called *Pneumocystis jiroveci*) and tumors (Kaposi Sarcoma) among homosexual men in California and New York. This was the beginning of the acquired immune deficiency syndrome (AIDS) pandemic. Initially, infection with the human immunodeficiency virus (HIV) appeared to be associated with homosexual activities, which led to the initial naming of gay-related immune deficiency syndrome (GRID). However, it soon became clear that heterosexual and direct blood contact could also transmit the newly recognized pathogen. Since then, HIV infection and AIDS have been spreading rapidly around the world, affecting millions of people and resulting in millions of deaths. In his speech at the 2003 International AIDS Conference in Paris, France, President Nelson Mandela declared HIV/AIDS the "greatest health crisis in human history."

In the last 30 years, achievements in the understanding, diagnosis, and treatment of HIV infection are considered among the most remarkable in medical history. Modern day antiretroviral therapy achieves control of the HIV infection and allows reconstitution of the immune system. HIV has become a chronic, manageable disease. However, to this date, HIV infection is not curable. Therefore, HIV prevention remains a key component in the fight against HIV and AIDS.

This chapter focuses on HIV transmission and prevention, HIV testing and early identification of HIV—topics, which are relevant in any primary care setting

G. Rieg, MD, FACP (✉)
Kaiser Permanente Medical Group, Medicine Department,
David Geffen School of Medicine at UCLA, Harbor City, CA, USA

Department of Medicine, Division of Infectious Diseases,
Kaiser Permanente South Bay Medical Center, 25965 So. Normandie Avenue, Harbor City,
CA 90710, USA
e-mail: grieg13@verizon.net

N.S. Skolnik et al. (eds.), *Sexually Transmitted Diseases: A Practical Guide for Primary Care*, Current Clinical Practice, DOI 10.1007/978-1-62703-499-9_7, © Springer Science+Business Media New York 2013

97

to counsel all patients and recognize and diagnose patients with HIV infections. As treatment becomes increasingly complex and ever changing, treatment guidelines are beyond the scope of this chapter but can be found at www.cdc.gov/HIV.

Prevalence and Incidence

The CDC estimates that 1.2 million people in the United States are infected with HIV [1]. It is estimated that 20 % of those are unaware of their HIV infection. The number of people living with HIV has increased in recent years due in part to enhanced HIV testing and improved treatment options leading to a prolonged life expectancy. It is expected that the number of people infected with HIV will continue to increase. Disturbingly, despite the efforts in prevention and the advances in HIV treatment, new HIV infections remain at a high level with approximately 50,000 Americans becoming newly infected with HIV each year.

Gay, bisexual, and other men who have sex with men are most severely affected by HIV infection accounting for 61 % of all new HIV infections in the latest available data from 2008 [1]. Ethnic minorities are disproportionally affected by HIV infection. Black Americans account for 46 % and Hispanic for 17 % of people living with HIV. The estimated rate of new HIV infection among Black American men is estimated to be 6.5 times as high as that of White American men and 2.5 times as high as that of Hispanic American men. Black American women are even more disproportionally affected by HIV with the new rate of HIV infection of Black American women being 15 times that of White American women and 3 times that of Hispanic/Latina women [1].

Transmission

Sexual contact is the most common route of HIV transmission. Worldwide, 75–85 % of HIV-infected individuals have been infected through sexual contact. The rate of HIV transmission through sexual contact is variable. Sexual transmission of HIV can occur in a single sexual encounter or might not occur for years in HIV-discordant couples (one HIV-infected partner and one HIV-negative partner) that have unprotected intercourse.

Sexual transmission of HIV via mucosal surfaces of the genital, oral, or rectal tract is influenced by multiple factors. In general, sexual transmission is dependent both on the concentration of HIV in genital secretions and on the susceptibility of the exposed partner. In infected people, HIV is present in the genital tract and in rectal secretions in women and men.

In women, although HIV can be recovered from the vagina, the glandular epithelium in the transformation zone between the columnar and squamous cells of the cervix appears to be a dominant source of HIV shedding. Concentrations of HIV from endocervical swabs have been found to be 2–3 times higher than from vaginal swabs [2, 3].

In men, HIV can be detected in seminal cells such as lymphocytes and monocytes as well as in seminal plasma (cell-free HIV) [4]. Although HIV DNA has been detected in sperm cells and their precursors [5], sperm itself appears to play no significant role in HIV transmission. Sperm cells do not possess CD4 receptors, which are the main cell receptor for HIV. Experience from assisted reproduction clinics—using washed and isolated spermatozoa for intrauterine insemination or for in vitro fertilization—washed sperms have not been associated with HIV transmission, confirming that spermatozoa alone do not play a significant role in HIV transmission [6, 7]. Vasectomy in men does not significantly affect HIV concentration in seminal secretion, suggesting that the majority of HIV shedding occurs distal of the vas deference [8].

To complicate matters, the genital tract can act as a separate compartment for HIV replication. The correlation between the HIV concentration in blood plasma and seminal secretion is only moderate [4, 8, 9]. Antiretroviral medication can achieve an undetectable HIV viral load in blood plasma, but this does not necessarily correlate with an undetectable viral level in the seminal secretions.

Rectal secretions have been found to have a significantly elevated of HIV concentration—in some circumstances even higher than HIV concentration in blood plasma and seminal fluid [10] contributing the high transmission risk with anal intercourse.

The exposed partner's susceptibility to HIV infection is also important in transmission efficacy. The partner's susceptibility depends on the presence of cells expressing CD4 receptors and chemokine surface receptors in the genital, oral, and/or rectal tissue [11]. The cells with CD4 receptors include CD4 T lymphocytes, Langerhans' cells, and other macrophages [12]. HIV-receptive cells have been found in the lamina propria of oral, cervicovaginal, foreskin, urethral, and rectal epithelia in primate models [12].

Different sexual practices are associated with different rates of transmission. The risk of HIV transmission per heterosexual contact in developed countries was estimated to be 0.04 % (four HIV transmissions per 10,000 sexual intercourse) in female-to-male transmission and 0.08 % (eight HIV transmissions in 10,000 sexual intercourse) in male-to-female transmission in a meta-analysis. The rate of HIV transmission in developing countries was estimated to be higher. Anal intercourse causes the highest risk of sexual HIV transmission with an estimated transmission rate of 1.7 % per act (170 HIV transmission per 10,000 sexual intercourse) [13]. An estimate of relative risk of different sexual acts is summarized in Table 7.1.

Several factors have been found to be associated with HIV transmission. The level of HIV viremia in the source patient is significantly associated with HIV transmission. In a study in Uganda, Gray and colleagues estimate the HIV transmission to be 0.23 % per act when the HIV serum level in the source is high (>38,500 viral load copies/mL), 0.13 % when the HV serum level is medium (1,700–28,499 viral load copies/mL), and 0.14 % when low (<1,700 viral load copies/mL) [15].

Sexually transmitted infections (STIs) increased the risk of HIV transmission. Especially genital ulcers in either partner increased the risk of HIV transmission by a factor of 5.3. On the other hand, circumcision has been found to decrease the risk

Table 7.1 Per act relative risk for acquisition of HIV

Sexual act					
Insertive oral	Receptive oral	Insertive vaginal	Insertive anal	Receptive vaginal	Receptive anal
1	2	10	13	20	100

Adapted from ref. [14]

HIV human immunodeficiency virus

of HIV transmission. Uncircumcised men are twice as likely to transmit/acquire HIV. Over time, stable HIV-discordant couples have a lower risk of transmitting HIV. In a given partnership, HIV transmission appears to occur within the early sexual contacts and is considerably less likely thereafter [16]. Consequently, a higher rate of HIV transmission should be expected in sexual assault cases. Sexual contact with multiple partners is associated with a higher risk of HIV transmission.

HIV Recognition and Testing

Given the high rate of new HIV infection in the United States as well as the large number of people already infected with HIV but not diagnosed yet, it is imperative to enhance recognition and testing of HIV. In contrary to previous HIV testing guidelines, the CDC recommended in 2006 that HIV testing should be part of routine medical care. In all health-care settings patients age 13–64 years old should be voluntarily tested for HIV as a routine test unless the HIV prevalence is less than 0.1 % in the population served. In addition, all patient initiating TB therapy and seeking treatment for STI should be tested. Repeat testing is recommended for patient at high risk for HIV infection such as injection-drug user and their sex partners, persons who exchange sex for money or drugs, sex partners of HIV-infected persons, men who have sex with men and persons who had more than one sex partner since their last HIV test. Consent and pre-/posttest counseling is not required by CDC guideline; however, the person tested for HIV need to be informed about the test and has the right to opt out [17].

All HIV diagnostic tests detect one or more molecules that comprise an HIV particle or detect antibodies that the host makes against the HIV particles [18]. The standard HIV test detects specific antibodies against HIV. Two different methods are used to detect antibodies. An enzyme-linked immunosorbent assay (ELISA) is used to screen for HIV-specific antibodies. The ELISA is more than 99 % sensitive and specific [19]. A Western blot assay, which detects HIV-specific antibodies, is used to confirm the HIV diagnosis. These two tests should be used in combination because false-negative and false-positive tests occur.

Newer HIV tests have been developed to either shorten the time period for a test result to be available ("rapid HIV test") or to improve patient convenience (oral HIV test, urine HIV test, HIV home kit test). Most of these rapid HIV tests must be performed by a trained laboratory technician and test results are available within 30 min.

In July 2012, the FDA approved the first over-the-counter home-use rapid HIV test (OraQuick In-Home HIV test). With this test, collect oral fluid sample by swabbing the upper and lower gums inside the mouth, then place that sample into a developer vial. Results can be read within 20–40 min. As with all rapid HIV tests, a positive result must be confirmed with the traditional standardized Western blot test.

Specific antibodies against HIV have some important clinical limitations. The ELISA and Western blot tests will be negative during the initial weeks after infection ("window period"), because antibodies are not usually detectable for 6–8 weeks. The time needed to perform the tests in the laboratory is also a disadvantage, as is the requirement for blood drawing in a clinical setting.

Patients often seek medical care with clinical symptoms of acute HIV seroconversion (during the "window period")—a frequently missed opportunity to diagnose newly acquired HIV infection [20]. Therefore, it is crucial to be aware of the symptoms of acute HIV infection. Acute retroviral syndrome (acute HIV infection syndrome) develops in 40–90 % of patients infected with HIV and starts approximately 2–6 weeks after exposure to HIV. It lasts for days to weeks, typically 14 days, but may persist up to 10 weeks. The development of specific antibodies against HIV marks the completion of seroconversion. Often, by the time of the onset of symptoms, the patient does not correlate the acute HIV conversion symptoms with the sexual encounter. Symptoms of an acute HIV infection are often mononucleosis-like and commonly include fever, rash, fatigue, pharyngitis, weight loss, night sweats, lymphadenopathy, myalgias, headache, nausea, and diarrhea. Mucosal ulcers (e.g., esophageal ulcers) can also be found. Neurological manifestations, such as aseptic meningitis, radiculopathy, and cranial nerve VII palsy, occur in some. Routine laboratory tests characteristically show leukopenia, thrombocytopenia, and elevated transaminases.

To diagnose acute HIV infection, HIV antibody tests may need to be repeated past the window period. In addition, nucleic acid tests for HIV may be used in consultation with an HIV/Infectious Disease specialist, to make a timely diagnosis of acute HIV infection. Counseling about safe sex practices to prevent transmission of HIV is obligate in patients with a high clinically suspicion for acute infection (Table 7.2).

Prevention

Prevention of HIV infection is the key intervention in fighting HIV infection and AIDS. Abstinence and mutual monogamy with a partner who has been tested and is known to be HIV-negative are the surest way to avoid HIV transmission. For sexually active persons with risk of HIV transmission, consistently and correctly used barrier methods (condoms) with or without pre-exposure therapy are efficient methods to reduce the risk for HIV transmission.

Male condoms are widely available and are the most commonly used barrier devices. Most male condoms are commonly made out of natural latex, but other materials are also used. Polyurethane condoms are considered an alternative to latex

Table 7.2 HIV testing recommendation (HIV prevalence >0.1 %)

At least one time testing (at health-care contact)
Everybody age 13–64 years old
Initiating tuberculosis therapy
Patient seeking STD testing/treatment
Repeat testing
Patient at high risk for HIV infection such as
Injection-drug user and their sex partners
Persons who exchange sex for money or drugs
Sex partners of HIV-infected persons
Men who have sex with men
Persons who had more than one sex partner since their last HIV test

condoms in patients with latex allergies. Natural condoms do not protect against HIV transmission and are not recommended for disease prevention, because they possess natural pores that may allow HIV to cross through the condom. Consistent and correct use to minimize breakage or slippage is essential to provide protection. In a meta-analysis of 12 cohort studies of HIV serodiscordant heterosexual couples, condom use—when used at every encounter—was estimated to be 87 % protective, which is comparable or slightly lower than its effectiveness to prevent pregnancy [21].

Data for anal intercourse are less robust. Anal intercourse is perceived as being associated with a higher breakage and slippage rate because of increased friction. Some European countries recommend the use of thicker/stronger condoms for anal intercourse. This recommendation has been based only on expert opinion; data to support the use of thicker and stronger condoms is sparse. A few small studies report a comparable breakage rate of standard and thicker condoms during anal intercourse [22, 23].

The female condom appears to be as protective as the male condom to prevent HIV transmission with correct and constant use (every time). It is less likely to break or leak when compared to the male condom [24].

There has been a great effort to evaluate microbicides in preventing HIV transmission—over 60 microbicides have been evaluated to prevent HIV infection. Microbicides are topical agents, which are applied to the vagina/rectum, may either directly inactivate HIV, prevent the attachment of HIV to target cells, inhibit HIV from entering and replicating in target cells, or prevent the dissemination of HIV from target cells. Targeting HIV entry is a preferred mechanism in the more advanced microbicides designed to prevent HIV transmission. While many studies could not show a protective effect of microbicides, the CAPRISA 004—a trial in South Africa using a 1 % tenofovir containing vaginal gel, showed an overall reduction of HIV acquisition by an estimated 39 % overall, and by 54 % in women with high gel adherence (>80 %) [25].

In July 2012, the FDA approved Truvada (a fixed dose combination of emtricitabine/tenofovir disoproxil fumarate) to reduce the risk of HIV infection in uninfected individuals. Truvada was initially approved in 2004 for the treatment of HIV infection in combination with other antiretroviral agents. Truvada is the first systemic HIV agent to be approved for pre-exposure prophylaxis (PrEP). Truvada was approved for use in individuals with high risk of HIV infection and in individuals who may engage in sexual activity with HIV-infected partners. In placebo-controlled studies, Truvada used in combination with condoms, reduced the risk of HIV infection in 42 % of men who have sex with men and 75 % in heterosexual individuals. However, it is imperative that individuals are compliant with the daily use of Truvada to achieve the protective effect of PrEP. Truvada as PrEP is to be used in combination with consistent and correct condom use and regular HIV testing and screening/treatment of STIs. This is part of the Risk Evaluation and Mitigation Strategy (REMS), which is a condition for use of Truvada as PrEP. Prior to initiating PrEP with Truvada, one must make sure that individuals are HIV-uninfected. In addition, individuals on PrEP require to be tested for HIV at least every 3 months in addition to undergoing frequent STI screening and treatment. There is a risk that HIV will develop resistance to the component of Truvada when the individuals would acquire HIV while taking the drug. Cost and possible toxicity of Truvada in routine clinical practice may limit the use of PrEP to a limited group of individuals.

Screening and aggressive treatment of STI other than HIV, especially STIs causing genital ulcers, will contribute to lower HIV transmission. Untreated genital ulcer disease doubles the risk of HIV transmission. Aggressive treatment of other STIs has been shown to lower the risk of HIV transmission by up to 40 % [26].

Postexposure prophylaxis (PEP) to prevent HIV infection after exposure is well established. Since 1996, the CDC published guidelines recommending antiretroviral therapy after exposure to HIV in an occupational setting (e.g., a health-care worker is accidentally exposed to blood of a known HIV-infected person) [27].

In 2005, the CDC published guidelines for PEP in nonoccupational settings (nPEP) (Fig. 7.1) [28]. Multidrug therapy for 28 days is recommended for people who present within 72 h of a nonoccupational exposure to blood, semen, vaginal secretions, rectal secretions, breast milk, or other body fluids that are contaminated with the blood of a person known to be HIV-infected. The earlier the prophylaxis is initiated, the better the chance of success. A history of the exposure, timing, and frequency of exposure, HIV status of the source as well as the exposed person and the risk for transmission needs to be assessed. Frequently exposed persons requiring frequent or even continuous prophylaxis should not receive PEP. If the status of the source person is not known, an attempt should be undertaken to test the source patient (if available). Prophylaxis for the exposed person can be initiated before the HIV test result of the source patient is known. If the HIV status of the source patient is unknown, a risk assessment of the source patient should be attempted (e.g., higher HIV prevalence among MSM, bisexual men, and iv drug users) and initiation of PEP should be determined on a case-by-case basis. The choice of HAART for PEP is based on the first-line recommendation by the Department of Health and Human Services for HIV-infected people. An Infectious Disease/HIV specialist should be consulted to assist in choosing the antiretroviral regimen. After initiating PEP, HIV antibody levels of the exposed patients should be determined at baseline, 4–6 weeks, 3, and 6 months. In addition, testing for hepatitis B and C and other STIs should be

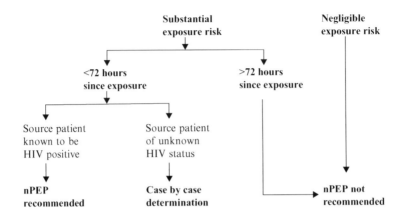

Substantial risk for HIV exposure:

Exposure of vagina, rectum, eye, mouth
Or other mucous membrane, non intact skin,
or percutaneous contact
with
blood, semen, vaginal secretion, rectal
secretion, breast milk, or any body fluid
contaminated with blood
when
the source patient is known to be HIV
positive status of the source

Negligible risk for HIV exposure

Exposure of vagina, rectum, eye,
mouth or other mucous membrane
intact or non-intact skin, or
percutaneous contact
with
urine, nasal secretions, saliva, sweat
or tears if not visibly contaminated
with blood
regardless
of the known or suspected HIV

Fig. 7.1 Nonoccupational postexposure prophylaxis

recommended and offered. Interaction with the person seeking PEP also provides an opportunity for safe sex counseling. Partner notification of the exposed person should be encouraged. If the exposed person becomes infected with HIV, partner notification is essential and required.

References

1. Centers for Disease Control and Prevention. HIV/AIDS surveillance report, Vol. 22; 2010. Atlanta, GA: US Department of Health and Human Services, Centers for Disease Control and Prevention. Available from: http://www.cdc.gov/hiv/stats/hasrlink.htm. Accessed 21 July 2012.
2. Clemetson DB, Moss GB, Willerford DM, et al. Detection of HIV DNA in cervical and vaginal secretions. Prevalence and correlates among women in Nairobi, Kenya. JAMA. 1993;269:2860–4.
3. Mostad SB, Overbaugh J, DeVange DM, et al. Hormonal contraception, vitamin A deficiency, and other risk factors for shedding of HIV-1 infected cells from the cervix and vagina. Lancet. 1997;350:922–7.

4. Vernazza PL, Eron JJ, Fiscus SA, Cohen MS. Sexual transmission of HIV: infectiousness and prevention. AIDS. 1999;13:155–66.

5. Bagasra O, Farzadegan H, Seshamma T, Oakes JW, Saah A, Pomerantz RJ. Detection of HIV-1 proviral DNA in sperm from HIV-1-infected men. AIDS. 1994;8:1669–74.

6. Bujan L, Pasquier C, Labeyrie E, Lanusse-Crousse P, Morucci M, Daudin M. Insemination with isolated and virologically tested spermatozoa is a safe way for human immunodeficiency type 1 virus-serodiscordant couples with an infected male partner to have a child. Fertil Steril. 2004;82:857–62.

7. Pasquier C, Daudin M, Righi L, et al. Sperm washing and virus nucleic acid detection to reduce HIV and hepatitis C virus transmission in serodiscordant couples wishing to have children. AIDS. 2000;14:2093–9.

8. Krieger JN, Nirapathpongporn A, Chaiyaporn M, et al. Vasectomy and human immunodeficiency virus type 1 in semen. J Urol. 1998;159:820–6.

9. Tachet A, Dulioust E, Salmon D, et al. Detection and quantification of HIV-1 in semen: identification of a subpopulation of men at high potential risk of viral sexual transmission. AIDS. 1999;13:823–31.

10. Zuckerman RA, Whittington WL, Celum CL, et al. Higher concentration of HIV RNA in rectal mucosa secretions than in blood and seminal plasma, among men who have sex with men, independent of antiretroviral therapy. J Infect Dis. 2004;190:156–61.

11. Dragic T, Litwin V, Allaway GP, et al. HIV-1 entry into CD4+ cells is mediated by the chemokine receptor CC-CKR-5. Nature. 1996;381:667–73.

12. Royce RA, Sena A, Cates Jr W, Cohen MS. Sexual transmission of HIV. N Engl J Med. 1997;336:1072–8.

13. Boily MC, Baggaley RF, Wang L, Masse B, White RG, Hayes RJ, et al. Heterosexual risk of HIV-1 infection per sexual act: systematic review and meta-analysis of observational studies. Lancet Infect Dis. 2009;9(2):118–29.

14. Varghese B, Maher JE, Peterman TA, Branson BM, Steketee RW. Reducing the risk of sexual HIV transmission: quantifying the per-act risk for HIV on the basis of choice of partner, sex act, and condom use. Sex Transm Dis. 2002;29:38–43.

15. Gray RH, Wawer MJ, Brookmeyer R, et al. Probability of HIV-1 transmission per coital act in monogamous, heterosexual, HIV-1-discordant couples in Rakai, Uganda. Lancet. 2001;357: 1149–53.

16. Downs AM, DeVincenzi I. Probability of heterosexual transmission of HIV: relationship to the number of unprotected sexual contacts. European Study Group in Heterosexual Transmission of HIV. J Acquir Immune Defic Syndr Hum Retrovirol. 1996;11:388–95.

17. Branson BM, Handsfield HH, Lampe MA, Janssen RS, Taylor AW, Lyss SB, et al.; Centers for Disease Control and Prevention (CDC). Revised recommendations for HIV testing of adults, adolescents, and pregnant women in health-care settings. MMWR Recomm Rep. 2006; 55(RR-14):1–17.

18. Iweala OI. HIV diagnostic tests: an overview. Contraception. 2004;70:141–7.

19. Mylonakis E, Paliou M, Lally M, Flanigan TP, Rich JD. Laboratory testing for infection with the human immunodeficiency virus: established and novel approaches. Am J Med. 2000;109:568–76.

20. Sudarshi D, Pao D, Murphy G, Parry J, Dean G, Fisher M. Missed opportunities for diagnosing primary HIV infection. Sex Transm Infect. 2008;84(1):14–6.

21. Davis KR, Weller SC. The effectiveness of condoms in reducing heterosexual transmission of HIV. Fam Plann Perspect. 1999;31:272–9.

22. Golombok S, Sheldon J. Evaluation of a thicker condom for use as a prophylactic against HIV transmission. AIDS Educ Prev. 1994;6:454–8.

23. Golombok S, Harding R, Sheldon J. An evaluation of a thicker versus a standard condom with gay men. AIDS. 2001;15:245–50.

24. Mitchell HS, Stephens E. Contraception choice for HIV positive women. Sex Transm Infect. 2004;80:167–73.

25. Karim AQ, Karim SSA, Frohlich JA, Grobler AC, Baxter C, Mansoor LE, et al. and on behalf of the CAPRISA 004 Trial Group. Effectiveness and safety of tenofovir gel, an antiretroviral microbicide, for the prevention of HIV infection in women. Science. 2010;329(5996):1168–74.
26. Grosskurth H, Mosha F, Todd J, et al. Impact of improved treatment of sexually transmitted diseases on HIV infection in rural Tanzania: randomised controlled trial. Lancet. 1995; 346:530–6.
27. Panlilio AL, Cardo DM, Grohskopf LA, Heneine W, Ross CS. Updated U.S. Public Health Service guidelines for the management of occupational exposures to HIV and recommendations for postexposure prophylaxis. MMWR. 2005;54(RR09):1–17.
28. Smith DK, Grohskopf LA, Black RJ, Auerback JD, Veronese F, Struble KA, et al. Antiretroviral postexposure prophylaxis after sexual, injection-drug use, or other nonoccupational exposure to HIV in the United States. MMWR. 2005;54(RR02):1–20.

Chapter 8
Syphilis

Carolyn M. Sutton

Introduction

Syphilis is a systemic infectious disease caused by sexual or congenital transmission of the bacterium *Treponema pallidum*. If left untreated, the infection progresses in stages with varied and often subtle clinical manifestations, which can result in serious and potentially life-threatening disease. With early treatment, few complications result [1]. Syphilis also facilitates the transmission of human immunodeficiency virus (HIV) [2].

Maternal primary and secondary (P&S) syphilis are associated with a 50 % probability of congenital syphilis and a 50 % rate of perinatal death [3]. Rates of both are lower in mothers with latent stage infection.

Epidemiology

The statistics for P&S syphilis reported in the United States in the early part of the twentieth century were very bleak. It was not until the introduction of antibiotics and broad public health measures in the 1940s that rates of syphilis dramatically declined. By 1957, the infection was almost entirely eliminated and rates remained manageable. In 2000, rates were at all low but began to steadily rise each year from 2001 to 2009. In 2010, the overall syphilis rate decreased for the first time in a decade and was down 1.6 % [4].

C.M. Sutton, MS, WHNP-BC, FAANP (✉)
Department of Obstetrics and Gynecology, University of Texas Southwestern
Medical Center at Dallas, Dallas, TX, USA

9710 Stone River Circle, Dallas, TX 75231, USA
e-mail: Carolyn.Sutton@UTSouthwestern.edu

N.S. Skolnik et al. (eds.), *Sexually Transmitted Diseases: A Practical Guide for Primary Care*, Current Clinical Practice, DOI 10.1007/978-1-62703-499-9_8,
© Springer Science+Business Media New York 2013

Today, rates remain highest in the South and in certain large urban centers in other parts of the country. Additionally, the rate among young black men has increased dramatically over the last 5 years and data also show a significant increase in infection among young black men who have sex with men (MSM) [5]. Fortunately, the national trends in P&S syphilis among reproductive-age women have decreased as have the pregnancy complication rates associated with the disease. In 2010, the rate of P&S among women was 1.2 cases per 100,000 women and the rate of congenital syphilis was 8.7 cases per 100,000 live births [5].

Risk Factors

Individuals at increased risk for contracting and transmitting syphilis in the United States include those who engage in high-risk behaviors, are diagnosed with other sexually transmitted infections (STIs), including HIV infection, MSM, commercial sex workers, exchange sex for drugs, are incarcerated, and those who are contacts of an individual with active syphilis [6]. The local incidence of syphilis in the community and the number of sex partners reported by an individual should be considered in identifying persons at high risk of infection. Lack of prenatal care, late or limited prenatal care, and maternal use of illicit drugs, including crack cocaine and methamphetamines, are associated with congenital syphilis [6].

Etiology

T. pallidum is an obligate human parasite and member of the family Spirochaetaceae. It is a thin, elongated organism with characteristic regularly round coils, with corkscrew mobility and the ability to flex at a 90° angle and replicate every 30–33 h [7]. The organism penetrates through the skin or mucosal tissue and spirochetemia occurs even before skin lesions develop or blood tests can detect infection. The mean incubation time is 21 days with a range of 10–90 days.

Transmission

T. pallidum is transmitted most commonly through direct contact with moist mucosal or cutaneous lesions during anal, vaginal, or oral-genital sex. Fomite transmission is not possible. It has been estimated that 3–10 % of individuals acquire the infection from a single sexual encounter with an infected partner.

Individuals are most infectious during the first year of infection, when the rate of transmission is 90 % [8]. Sexual transmission drops dramatically after that; by the second year, transmission is 5 %, and by the end of the fourth year, syphilis can no longer be contracted by sexual contact. In untreated populations, 50–75 % of sex partners of people diagnosed with primary or secondary syphilis are infected.

Maternal-fetal or vertical transmission can occur either through transplacental spread or at the time of delivery from direct contact with syphilitic lesions. Transplacental infection generally occurs after 18 weeks of gestation because of the relative immunocompetence before that gestational age [6]. However, fetal infection risks are highest in women with early syphilis.

Other means of transmission are very rare, but include transfusion and accidental direct inoculation. Indirect evidence suggests that needle sharing by intravenous drug users may contribute to some cases [9].

Natural Course: Four Stages

Primary Stage

Primary syphilis, the earliest stage of the disease, is defined by the lesion that appears at the site of the inoculation—the chancre. This is a painless, ulcerated lesion with a raised border, and an indurated and clear base that is teeming with infectious treponemes. The most common site for the chancre is the genital area but extragenital sites may also be affected. A solitary lesion is common but multiple chancres can occur in up to 30 % of cases. Painless inguinal lymphadenopathy is frequently present. The primary chancre heals spontaneously in 3–6 weeks after appearance.

Secondary Stage

The secondary stage represents dissemination of *T. pallidum* throughout the body; therefore, any organ can be potentially infected. This highly infectious stage occurs simultaneously with or up to 6 months after the healing of the primary chancre. Symptoms that may appear in this stage include low-grade fever, malaise, and headache; generalized and non-tender lymphadenopathy, a generalized rash that is also present on the soles of the feet and the palms of the hands; painless mucus patches in the oral cavity or genital tract, condylomata lata in warm and moist areas; and, alopecia. Organ systems such as the kidney, liver, joints, and central nervous system may also be involved. Untreated symptoms of secondary syphilis will spontaneously disappear in 3–12 weeks.

Latent Stage

Latency follows resolution of secondary syphilis. This is a period of time when there are no clinical manifestations of the disease but serologic tests for detection of specific antibodies to *T. pallidum* remain positive. Early latency includes the first year of infection. The late latency phase begins 1 year after infection or when the duration of the infection is unknown. In the late latent phase, people are not contagious by sexual transmission but the spirochete may still be transplacentally transmitted to a fetus. Without treatment, one-third progress and develop tertiary syphilis.

Tertiary Stage

The tertiary stage may begin as early as 1 year after infection or at any time during an infected person's lifetime. Today, the clinical symptoms of tertiary syphilis are rarely seen. When present, the clinical expression depends on which of the specific complications develop. Treponemes invade the central nervous system, cardiovascular system, eyes, skin, and other organs.

Neurosyphilis occurs when *T. pallidum* invades the central nervous system early in the course of the infection. It is divided into early and late forms. Spontaneous clearance of the spirochete occurs in 75 % of cases; with adequate antibiotic treatment of early infection, few immunocompetent individuals do not clear. However, those who have persistent spirochetes in the central nervous system are at risk for symptomatic neurosyphilis. Overall, in untreated populations, 4–9 % of cases developed into early neurosyphilis. Early neurosyphilis coexists with primary or secondary infections and is usually asymptomatic. The cerebrospinal fluid, cerebral blood vessels, and meninges are often involved, but the brain and spinal cord are usually spared. Meningeal syphilis presents with headache, stiff neck, nausea, and vomiting with or without cranial nerve involvement. Meningovascular syphilis causes focal ischemia or stroke. On the other hand, late neurosyphilis affects the meninges and brain or spinal cord; it develops in 4–14 % of cases of untreated early neurosyphilis. Tabes dorsales (locomotor ataxia) is a spinal cord disorder with sensory ataxia (including blindness because of optic atrophy), lightening pains, and bladder and bowel dysfunction.

Gummatous disease is a particularly disfiguring manifestation of tertiary syphilis. It affects 15 % of untreated cases and develops 1–46 years after initial infection. The gummatous lesion is most often nodular and characterized by granulomatous inflammation and necrosis. The size of these benign but highly tissue-destructive lesions range from microscopic to many centimeters in diameter and may be found in any tissue or organ. They are, however, most commonly found in soft tissue and bone. Although spirochetes may not be detectable in biopsy specimens, the treponemal serological tests will be reactive in the presence of gummatous disease.

After the introduction of antibiotics, cardiovascular syphilis became extremely rare. Today it is estimated that only 10 % of the untreated cases of syphilis will develop serious cardiac involvement. Because syphilis affecting the cardiovascular system only manifests clinically in the tertiary stage of the disease, the onset of symptoms may be delayed for 20–30 years after the initial infection. Cardiovascular syphilis may lead to aortic aneurysms, aortic insufficiency, coronary stenosis, and myocarditis.

Diagnostic Testing

T. pallidum cannot be cultured. In initial disease, dark-field microscopy of exudate from the lesion is a reliable diagnostic method used to confirm the presence of spirochetes. Incident light through a microscope fitted with polarizing lenses allows the viewer to identify the corkscrew morphology of treponemes as white against a black background. Exudate for dark-field microscopy can be collected from the base of the chancre that has been cleaned with saline. In the absence of dark-field microscopy, direct fluorescent antibody stains of the exudates can also be used to identify *T. pallidum*. Specificity of these tests is highly dependent on the skill of the microscopist. Most clinicians do not have the equipment (dark-field microscope) or laboratory support to perform these tests.

Serological testing for antibodies to *T. pallidum* forms the basis of diagnostic testing in the United States. The initial test used is the one that tests quantitatively for the presence of nontreponemal antibodies, using either the Venereal Disease Research Laboratory (VDRL) or the reactive plasma reagin (RPR) tests. Nontreponemal tests are used to test patients for the presence of antibodies to another protein, cardiolipin, which develop and rise in titer following infection.

It must be remembered that the test requires that the patient has had time and ability to mount an antibody response to the infection. In early primary syphilis, antibody levels may be too low to detect and nontreponemal tests may be nonreactive. Only 30 % of individuals infected with primary stage syphilis will become serologically positive 1 week after appearance of the chancre, but 90 % will be positive after 3 weeks [7]. Nontreponemal tests are 78–89 % sensitive in primary syphilis, but are almost 100 % sensitive in secondary syphilis. In late syphilis, titers decline and previously reactive results revert to nonreactive in 25 % of cases, and test sensitivity averages only 70 %. Therefore, nontreponemal tests cannot establish a definitive diagnosis of syphilis, especially in the early or latent stages of the disease. False-positive results may occur with nontreponemal tests because other disease processes can modify cardiolipin causing the same antibody development [10] This may occur with autoimmune disease, intravenous drug use, vaccination, pregnancy, HIV, pneumonia, hepatitis, hepatic disease (mononucleosis), tuberculosis, bacterial endocarditis, and other spirochetal malarial or rickettsial infections [11].

Because nontreponemal tests are associated with high sensitivity and low specificity, specific treponemal tests, such as fluorescent treponemal antibody-absorption (FTA-ABS) test or *T. pallidum* passive-particle agglutination (TP-PA) test are used to confirm the diagnosis of syphilis in patients with a reactive nontreponemal test. These confirmatory assays have high sensitivity and the specificity rate is 98 %. However, some false positives can occur with these tests in the presence of certain acute and chronic diseases [10]. Therefore, when used sequentially, the positive predictive value of the combined tests is high and reactive results are likely to represent true infection [4].

Diagnosis

In early infection, a presumptive diagnosis of syphilis can be made based on the patient's history and findings on physical examination. Specific tests, such as dark-field microscopy, are more secure, but often not available. A positive treponemal-specific test (in the absence of prior infection) can be confirmatory even if the nontreponemal test is negative.

After the initial infection, however, diagnosis requires that both the nontreponemal and treponemal tests be reactive. Occasionally, a low titer reactive result may be obtained, indicating either new infection or a false-positive. Recent infection can be confirmed by documenting an increase in titer of the nontreponemal test over time. Because the accuracy of the test may vary by a dilution, the increase must be two dilutions or a fourfold increase on titers (such as 1:8–1:32) to demonstrate a clinically significant difference between tests. The CDC cautions that when serially monitoring patients for diagnosis, the same nontreponemal test (RPR or VDRL) should be used and preferably, the tests should be processed by the same laboratory. Some HIV-infected patients may have unusual serological test results over time, so other modalities, including biopsy or direct microscopy may be needed.

Neurosyphilis may occur at any stage of infection with *T. pallidum*. Therefore, any syphilitic person presenting with neurological complaints, such as stiff neck, severe persistent headache, or hearing compromise should undergo lumbar puncture and cerebrospinal fluid evaluation using a combination of tests including cell count, protein, and VDRL-CSF with or without FTA-ABS testing. Those with visual complaints should be evaluated for uveitis using a slit-lamp examination.

In the tertiary stage of syphilis, the sensitivity of nontreponemal tests ranges from 71 to 73 %. Treponemal-specific tests are positive in this stage with a sensitivity of 94–96 %.

All patients diagnosed with syphilis should be tested for HIV and for other STIs. In areas of high HIV prevalence, HIV tests should be repeated in 3 months.

Treatment

The CDC-recommended preferred treatment for syphilis in non-pregnant and non-HIV-infected individuals is intramuscular administration of penicillin G. The preparation(s) used (i.e., benzathine, aqueous procaine, or aqueous crystalline), the dosage, and the length of treatment depend on the stage and clinical manifestations of disease [11]. The most important property is that bacteriocidal levels of the medication are maintained for several weeks to kill the slowly metabolizing *T. pallidum*.

No alternatives to penicillin have been proved effective for treatment of syphilis during pregnancy. Within 24 h of treatment, up to 60 % of cases have a Jarisch–Herxheimer reaction, which includes fever, myalgia, headache, malaise, sore throat, and vasodilatation with mild hypotension and tachycardia [12]. The reaction results from an antigen overload, which is more likely to occur in early syphilis. It may result from prostaglandin release or as an immune response. This reaction can induce early labor or fetal distress [12].

Follow-Up

Treatment failure is possible with any regimen. The CDC recommends that patients should be reexamined clinically and serologically 6 and 12 months following treatment. More frequent evaluations may be prudent if follow-up is uncertain. HIV-infected patients require more frequent and prolonged follow-up intervals (3, 6, 9, 12, and 24 months). Patients with latent syphilis should have quantitative nontreponemal tests repeated at 6, 12, and 24 months. Those with neurosyphilis need CSF tests done every 6 months until their cell count normalizes.

It is expected that titers of nontreponemal tests will decline by at least two titers (fourfold) to demonstrate initial response. Over time, most successfully treated patients will revert to undetectable levels of nontreponemal titers. The treponemal-specific antibodies generally remain positive throughout life.

Patients with persistent or recurrent signs or symptoms or who sustain a fourfold increase in nontreponemal test titer over the baseline titer should be considered to be treatment failures or re-infected. They need to be retreated and reevaluated for HIV infection.

Partner Notification and Reporting Requirements

It is important to identify and treat any possible sexual contacts of patients with syphilis. In patients with primary syphilis, all contacts for 3 months before the appearance of the chancre should be evaluated clinically and with serological tests. In patients with secondary syphilis, contacts for 6 months before the onset of the signs associated with secondary syphilis should be evaluated clinically and serologically. In patients with early latent syphilis and no history or signs suggestive of primary or secondary stage disease, contacts for 12 months prior should be evaluated clinically and serologically. Persons with known exposure to a patient with early syphilis within the previous 3 months can be infected and seronegative and should, therefore, be treated presumptively. Syphilis is a reportable disease in all states and territories.

Special Issues

Syphilis in Pregnancy

Antepartum syphilis produces serious adverse outcomes for the pregnant woman and her fetus. Transplacental transmission is the most common acquisition route for the neonate. However, infection may also follow after contact with spirochetes through contact with lesions at delivery [3]. Maternal syphilis has been associated with obstetric complications, such as hydramnios, abortion, and preterm delivery, and fetal complications such as fetal syphilis, hydrops, prematurity, fetal distress, and stillbirth [3]. The frequency of congenital syphilis varies with both the stage and duration of maternal infection; the highest incidence occurs in neonates born to mothers with early syphilis and the lowest incidence occurs with late latent disease. If the maternal infection is acquired within 4 years of the pregnancy, infection of the fetus occurs in more than 70 % of cases [3].

Syphilis screening is recommended for all women at the first prenatal visit. For women at high risk for syphilis, screening should be repeated at 32 weeks and again at delivery [4]. In addition, any woman who delivers a stillborn after 20 weeks gestation should be tested for syphilis.

Only penicillin should be used to treat pregnant women. Other agents may eradicate the maternal infection, but they do not reliably treat the fetus [13]. Therefore, a pregnant woman who is allergic to penicillin should undergo desensitization in a hospital setting and then be treated with the penicillin regimen that is appropriate for the stage of syphilis infection [14].

HIV and Syphilis

Epidemiological studies demonstrate that a history of sexually transmitted diseases, including syphilis, is associated with an increased risk for HIV infection, and that genital ulcers caused by sexually transmitted diseases are cofactors for acquiring HIV infection [15, 16]. Isolated case reports have suggested that coexistent HIV infection may alter the natural history of syphilis and the dosage or duration of treatment required to cure syphilis [17]. It is suggested that impairment of both cell-mediated and humeral immunity by HIV limits the host's defenses against *T. pallidum*, thereby altering the clinical manifestations or natural course of the disease [18].

Standard serological tests appear to be accurate and reliable for the diagnosis of syphilis and the evaluation of treatment response in HIV-infected individuals, although additional testing may be needed to rule out some of the complications of advanced disease, such as neurosyphilis. More frequent and prolonged follow-ups are also necessary.

HIV-infected persons with primary, secondary, or latent syphilis should be treated with the same regimens as a noninfected individual, but it is recommended that those with late latent or syphilis of unknown duration have an analysis of the cerebrospinal fluid before initiation of therapy [18]. These persons should be managed by an HIV infection expert

References

1. Eccleston K, Collins L, Higgins SP. Primary syphilis. Int J STD AIDS. 2008;19(3):145–51.
2. Musher DM. Early syphilis. In: Holmes KK, Sparling PF, Mardh PA, Lemon SM, Stamm WE, Piot P, Wasserheit JW, editors. Sexually transmitted diseases. 4th ed. New York, NY: McGraw Hill; 2009.
3. Creasy R, Resnik R, Iams J, et.al., editors. Maternal and fetal infections. In: Creasy and Resnik maternal-fetal medicine. 6th ed. Philadelphia: Saunders; 2009
4. United States Preventive Services Task Force. Screening for syphilis infection: recommendation statement. Ann Fam Med. 2009;15(10):705–9.
5. Centers for Disease Control and Prevention. Sexually transmitted disease surveillance. Atlanta: U.S. Department of Health and Human Services; 2010.
6. Cunningham G, Leveno K, Bloom S, et.al., editors. Sexually transmitted diseases. In: Williams obstetrics. 23rd ed. New York: McGraw Hill; 2010.
7. Garnett GP, Aral SO, Hoyle DV, Cates Jr W, Anderson RM. The natural history of syphilis: Implications for the transmission dynamics and control of infection. Sex Transm Dis. 1997;24:185–200.
8. Magnuson HJ, Thomas EW, Olansky S, Kaplan BI, De Mello L, Cutler JC. Inoculation of syphilis in human volunteers. Medicine (Baltimore). 1956;35:33–82.
9. Nelson KE, Vlahov D, Cohn S, et al. Sexually transmitted diseases in a population of intravenous drug users: association with seropositivity to the human immunodeficiency virus (HIV). J Infect Dis. 1991;164:457–63.
10. Carlsson B, Hanson HS, Wasserman J, Brauner A. Evaluation of the fluorescent treponemal antibody-absorption (FTA-Abs) test specificity. Acta Derm Venereol. 1991;71(4):306–11.
11. Centers for Disease Control and Prevention. Primary and secondary syphilis—United States. MMWR Morb Mortal Wkly Rep. 2010;59(14):413–7.
12. Myles T, Elam F, Park-Hwang E, Nguyen T. The Jarisch-Herxheimer reaction and fetal monitoring changes in pregnant women treated for syphilis. Obstet Gynecol. 1998;92(5):859–64.
13. Wendel Jr GD, Sheffield JS, Hollier LM, Hill JB, Ramsey PS, Sanchez PJ. Treatment of syphilis in pregnancy and prevention of congenital syphilis. Clin Infect Dis. 2002;35:S200–9.
14. Wendel Jr GO, Stark BJ, Jamison RB, Melina RD, Sullivan TJ. Penicillin allergy and desensitization in serious infections during pregnancy. N Engl J Med. 1985;312:1229–32.
15. Darrow W, Echenberg D, Jaffe H, et al. Risk factors for human immunodeficiency virus (HIV) infections in homosexual men. Am J Public Health. 1987;77:479–83.
16. Greenblatt RM, Lukehart SA, Plummer FA, et al. Genital ulceration as a risk factor for human immunodeficiency virus infection. AIDS. 1988;2:47–50.
17. Johns D, Tierney M, Felsenstein D. Alteration in the natural history of neurosyphilis by concurrent infection with the human immunodeficiency virus. N Engl J Med. 1987;316:1569–72.
18. Bowen DL, Lane HC, Fauci AS. Immunopathogenesis of the acquired immunodeficiency syndrome. Ann Intern Med. 1985;103:704–9.

Chapter 9
Trichomoniasis

Anne Moore

Introduction

Trichomonas vaginalis was first discovered by Donnéin (1836). Today, it is responsible for 25 % of all cases of clinically diagnosed vaginitis. More than half of infected women and nearly 90 % of infected men are asymptomatic, which increases the reservoir of people spreading the infection. Trichomoniasis increases the risks of human immunodeficiency virus (HIV) transmission and HIV acquisition.

Fast Facts

- There are five million new infections with *T. vaginalis* in the United States each year.
- The routine diagnostic test—microscopic evaluation of a vaginal specimen—detects only 50–60 % of infections.
- Treatment of the nonpregnant woman and her partner is necessary even if they had no symptoms.
- Some strains of *T. vaginalis* are now resistant to metronidazole and require higher dose therapy with metronidazole or treatment with tinidazole.

A. Moore, DNP, APN, FAANP (✉)
School of Nursing, Vanderbilt University, Nashville, TN, USA

456 Deer Ridge Lane, Nashville, TN 37221, USA
e-mail: anne.moore@Vanderbilt.Edu

N.S. Skolnik et al. (eds.), *Sexually Transmitted Diseases: A Practical Guide for Primary Care*, Current Clinical Practice, DOI 10.1007/978-1-62703-499-9_9,
© Springer Science+Business Media New York 2013

Prevalence and Incidence

Trichomoniasis is the second most common sexually transmitted infection (STI) after human papillomavirus. Because this STI is not a reportable disease, data regarding actual numbers of cases remain elusive. However, it has been estimated that there are five million new cases in the United States each year, which is more than the sum of all cases of *chlamydia* and gonococcal infections [1, 2]. The World Health Organization estimates that there are 173 million new infections worldwide per year [3].

Prevalence rates for trichomoniasis infections with *T. vaginalis* vary with different types of clinical settings. For example, Soper reported that studies in sexually transmitted disease clinics found that between 15 and 54 % of women in those sites had culture or polymerase chain reaction (PCR) evidence of trichomonal infection, 43 % of patients in substance abuse facilities, 47 % of prison inmates, 10–13 % of women in student health, and 11–22 % of HIV-infected or at-risk women were found to have trichomonal infections [4].

Earlier studies suggested that 6–15 % of asymptomatic women undergoing annual Pap smears had *T. vaginalis* [5]. In contrast to other STIs, such as *chlamydia* and gonorrhea, peak years of prevalence for trichomoniasis occur later in life—among 20- to 46-year-olds. There is generally a longer duration of infectiousness and a high level of asymptomatic infections, especially in men.

Risk Factors

Risk factors for trichomoniasis include all the risks generally associated with STI acquisition—multiple or new partners, nonuse of barrier method of contraception, young age, minority member, lower socioeconomic status, and other STIs. Chlamydial infection is a particularly high risk factor; up to 30 % of women with chlamydial cervicitis also have trichomoniasis.

Infectivity and Transmission

The primary mode of transmission of *T. vaginalis* is through sexual contact. Transmission by fomites is possible, but is rarely the cause of a symptomatic infection. An inoculum of at least 10,000 organisms is needed to establish a clinically significant infection; fomites are usually not able to deliver that large a deposit of organisms. Male-to-female transmission rates are higher than female-to-male rates; about 85 % of exposed women will contract the infection. Female-to-male transmission rates are more variable, but may be as high as 70 % within 48 h of exposure [4]. Incubation period varies from 4 to 28 days [6].

Etiology

T. vaginalis is a unicellular, anaerobic, flagellated protozoan. The organism was first described in 1836 by Donné.. The usual size range of this parasite is 5–15 μ long, but it can grow to 30 μ. It has a short undulating membrane, which extends only half way to the end of the body. The organism relies heavily on the host to obtain all nutrients as preformed molecules; it has little or no biosynthetic capability of its own. It even lacks mitochondria. *T. vaginalis* resembles anaerobic bacteria more than eukaryotic behavior in that it ferments large amounts of carbohydrates into carbon dioxide and hydrogen gases, causing bubbles. Its presence in the vaginal vault changes the vaginal microbiology—the lactobacilli disappear and anaerobic bacteria predominant. *T. vaginalis* swims freely in the vaginal discharge but can also attach to the vaginal wall. The cell membranes of the parasite and those of the host interdigitate. Trichomonads adhere to vaginal and cervical epithelial cells. *T. vaginalis* also infects the urethra, Skene's glands, and Bartholin glands. The organism does not invade into the underlying tissues but precipitates an intense inflammatory response locally [7].

This inflammatory response is responsible not only for the characteristic clinical and laboratory findings of leukocytosis but it also explains the increased vulnerability of people infected with *T. vaginalis* have to acquiring HIV. HIV can gain ready access through disruptions in the epithelium to HIV target cells, such as CD4-bearing lymphocytes and macrophages concentrated in the area in response to the *T. vaginalis* infection. Trichomoniasis also increases the infectivity of HIV-infected individuals [8, 9]. Treatment of *T. vaginalis* in HIV-infected women decreases cell-free HIV-1 virus by 4.2-fold in the vagina. Similarly, trichomoniasis-infected men with HIV have a sixfold higher concentration of HIV RNA in their seminal plasma than those without trichomonal infections [10].

Clinical Manifestations

Half of women infected with *T. vaginalis* are asymptomatic, but about 30 % of these women will develop symptoms when they are followed for 6 months [11]. Women who develop symptoms may complain of increased vaginal discharge, which has a green hue, frothy appearance, and foul odor. The odor may not be because of the original trichomonal infection, but may result from concomitant bacterial vaginosis. Women may also have complaints of urinary frequency, dysuria, dyspareunia, and/or postcoital spotting. Dysuria and frequency may be caused by a urethral infection; dyspareunia and postcoital spotting generally result from the inflamed and friable cervix. Some women may note vulvar irritation, pruritus, or edema.

Only about 10 % of men infected with *T. vaginalis* develop symptoms. Latif et al. suggested that men may be more resistant to infection or may be able to clear the infection without developing symptoms or treatment [12]. It is unlikely that men are resistant to infection, because a serological survey found that men and women were as likely to have antibodies to *T. vaginalis* [13]. This high level of asymptomatic infection in men is important to emphasize when counseling women who are diagnosed with trichomoniasis; they should expect that their sex partners will deny having symptoms. Symptoms in men are nonspecific. They may have urethral discharge and/or dysuria. More severe symptoms are more likely to be reported in cases in which the infection involves the prostate or seminal vesicles. One study found trichomoniasis in 5.5 % of men with nongonococcal urethritis. Interestingly, the men with *T. vaginalis* as a cause of nongonococcal urethritis had experienced symptoms for nearly twice as long than men with other etiologies [12]. The discharge these men experienced was also different from other STI-related urethral discharges; it was characterized as a white, watery discharge with tiny clumps of material. When these clumps were examined microscopically, large numbers of epithelial cells with some white cells were seen. Interestingly, the diagnosis of *T. vaginalis* also occurred in men who were treated for laboratory-confirmed cases of gonococcal urethritis, suggesting that initially the men had dual infections. Prostatitis with or without epididymitis is an uncommon complication. Therefore, other STIs should be ruled out before attributing these complications to trichomonal infection.

On physical examination, an infected woman may have copious amounts of frothy discharge at her introitus with erythema and some edema in the vestibule and surrounding labia. The vaginal vault may be coated with gray or yellow–green-colored frothy discharge, which often pools in the upper vault. The bubbles in the discharge, which are characteristic of this infection, result from the metabolism of carbohydrates into carbon dioxide and hydrogen gases. However, frothiness was found in only 12–34 % of cases in Gardener and Duke's series [14]. Wiping away the discharge from the cervix, the portio may seem to have an injected, edematous appearance speckled with clusters of petechia (punctate mucosal hemorrhages), which has classically been described as a "strawberry" or "flea-bitten" cervix. These petechiae are best seen with colposcopic magnification. The cervix may be quite friable, but in the absence of other STIs, there should not be cervical motion tenderness.

Testing and Diagnosis

T. vaginalis can be isolated in urine, semen, and vaginal discharge. The standard diagnostic test is microscopic examination of vaginal discharge. Collecting and handling of the specimen are critically important in improving the sensitivity of the wet-mount test. The classic technique of placing a drop of the vaginal secretions directly onto a slide and mixing in some normal saline, then trapping the specimen under a cover slide is most effective when the specimen is promptly examined. Any substantial delay in examining the specimen (e.g., when other specimens are collected, bimanual exam is performed, and the patient is counseled about physical findings) allows the specimen to dry out. After drying, the protozoan loses its characteristic pear shape and becomes rounded. In this shape, it is easy to overlook it in sheets of similar shaped (but smaller) leukocytes, which are present in abundance. Twenty percent of wet mounts initially positive for *T. vaginalis* become negative within 10 min, and 87 % disappear within 2 h. In order to retain the pear-shape morphology of *T. vaginalis*, the clinician should suspend the vaginal specimen in a test tube with normal saline that has no preservatives. When it is time to do microscopy, a drop of the dilute specimen can be placed onto the slide for examination. At room temperature, *T. vaginalis* may lose its rapid motion, but if the pear-shaped organism is observed, a slow undulation will be seen. This dilution of the specimen also allows separation of the epithelial cells so that their borders are easier to examine to rule out concomitant bacterial vaginosis.

The sensitivity of the microscopic examination of the vaginal discharge varies from 42 to 92 % [15], with most studies reporting sensitivities of 50–60 % [16]. The variation seen is a function not only of the technique used but also the time spent searching for *T. vaginalis* in the microscopic sample. Sweet reported that experienced technicians can detect 80 % of cases, but that the sensitivity drops to 50 % when the test is performed by busy clinicians [15]. Ledger reports even lower accuracy. He found considerable errors in diagnoses; only 51.2 % of patients with culture proven infection were detected on microscopy and 25 % of women diagnosed with trichomoniasis microscopically did not have the infection on culture [17].

There are two FDA-cleared tests for *trichomonas* in women: the OSOM *Trichomonas* Rapid test (Genzyme Diagnostics, Cambridge, MA), which uses an immunochromatographic capillary flow dipstick technology and a nucleic acid probe test called the Affirm VP II System (Becton Dickinson), which uses synthetic probes for detection of *T. vaginalis*, bacterial vaginosis, and *Candida* from a single vaginal swab. These tests have greater than 83 % sensitivity and specificity greater than 97 %, compared to culture.

Other techniques that have been tested for diagnosis of *T. vaginalis* infection include monoclonal antibody staining of direct specimens [18]. This technology has been shown to have a 92 % sensitivity overall and a 77 % sensitivity in women with negative microscopy. Monoclonal antibody staining provides rapid answers; however, the need for specific reagents and high-quality microscopy rules this out as an office-based procedure [19]. PCR tests have been developed that are more sensitive than cultures and can distinguish *T. vaginalis* from other trichomonal species. The test is too expensive for routine use at this time. Lobo et al. reported that the sensitivity of traditional testing modalities, when compared with PCR, is lower than generally recognized.

For example, when compared with PCR, culture is only 79 % as sensitive, wet mounts are 66 % as sensitive, and Pap smear sensitivity was 61 % [20].

The gold standard technique for diagnosis has been culture; the sensitivities of other tests are measured against it. Culture is straightforward, but special culture media are needed. The two most commonly used media are Diamond or Kupferberg media, but laboratory support for processing cultures is frequently not available. Products such as InPouch TV™ (Biomed Diagnostics, San Jose, CA) have been developed to combine culture and microscopy [21]. Generally, only 1000–10,000 organisms are necessary for an infection to be detected on culture. Negative results will not be available for up to 7 days, but positive results may be available earlier. The best specimen to culture in women is material from the vaginal vault. In men, urethral pus or a spun-down urine specimen (urine sediment) may be cultured.

In general, the conventional Pap smear has been found to be a poor diagnostic test of trichomoniasis. It has low sensitivity (52–67 %) and a low specificity (83–99 %), even when the smear is prepared with a vital strain, such as acridine orange [15]. Although it is acknowledged that conventional Pap smears are not useful in screening women for this infection, clinicians are often left with the challenge of how best to manage women whose Pap smear reports the presence of *T. vaginalis*. Today it is recognized that asymptomatic infections in nonpregnant women warrant treatment, but the accuracy of the Pap smear must be questioned. In one study comparing various test procedures, cytological smear were interpreted as positive in 56 % of the women who actually had infection detected by other methods, but another 1 % of the population tested were read as positive and 3 % were read as "suspicious" when they had negative cultures. The authors found a positive predictive value of only 69 % [18]. For many women the issue of having an infection, which is probably sexually transmitted, is important to their relationships. Therefore, the correct management of an asymptomatic woman with an isolated Pap smear reporting *T. vaginalis* is controversial. Some argue that because trichomoniasis is an important STI and treatment is not associated with much cost or side effects, women should be offered treatment based on the Pap smear results alone. This automatic treatment is a reasonable approach for women who are in high-prevalence populations or who are at higher personal risk for having the infection. One example would be the woman who has been recently diagnosed with *chlamydia* and her Pap smear reported *T. vaginalis*. For lower risk women, there is more conflict. This is because the traditional diagnostic test used—the wet mount—is very insensitive. The argument is that if a woman really had trichomoniasis (suggested by her Pap smear), there would be a 40–50 % of missing it with a microscopic evaluation of her vaginal discharge. One solution would be to seek the woman's counsel about her willingness to be treated with no further work-up. If she prefers to have more information, perform a wet mount and treat the positive results. If her wet mount is negative, perform more sensitive testing (such as a culture).

Liquid-based Papanicolaou cervical cytology testing may improve the detection of *T. vaginalis* compared with conventional Pap smear. One study found that compared to culture, liquid-based Pap testing had a sensitivity of 61.4 % (virtually the same as conventional tests) but an improved specificity of 99.4 %. This improved the positive predictive value to 96.4 % [16].

In men, diagnosis is even more challenging. It is difficult to identify *T. vaginalis* in either a centrifuged deposit of urine or urethral discharge suspended in normal saline. In one study, only 50 % of men with the infection had it detected on first microscopic examination. Wet-mount microscopic studies of urethral samples had only 30 % sensitivity and urethral cultures detected only 60 % of infections [22]. PCR has the ability to detect 4 times more infections than combined cultures of urethra and urethral swabs. Culture testing of urethral swabs, urine, and semen is required for optimal sensitivity. The intrinsic insensitivity of tests of men is another reason that male sex partners of infected women need to be treated on an epidemiological basis—even if they have no evidence of personal infection. Patients with trichomoniasis should be evaluated for other STIs.

Treatment

Metronidazole has been the drug of choice for the treatment of infections with *T. vaginalis* since 1960 [23]. The Center for Disease Control and Prevention recommendations for treatment of uncomplicated trichomoniasis have remained constant for the last several years. The recommended regimen is metronidazole 2 g or tinidazole 2 g orally in a single dose. Metronidazole single-dose therapy has a cure rate of 90–95 % [24]. Tinidazole's cure rate is 86–100 %. Tinidazole has more complete tissue penetration and lower minimum lethal concentrations than metronidazole [25]. Lower doses of metronidazole have been studied in an attempt to decrease gastrointestinal side effects. The 1.5-mg dose was roughly equivalent to the 2 mg dose, and had fewer side effects, but even lower doses were associated with unacceptably high failure rates [26]. The alternative recommendation of metronidazole 500 mg orally twice a day for 7 days is thought to be equivalent and to have similar side effect rates as single dose therapy [27], but is associated with lower compliance rates. Incomplete use of 7-day treatments has resulted in the emergence of strains of *T. vaginalis* that are more resistant to metronidazole. Oral systemic therapies are needed because *T. vaginalis* can be sequestered in the Bartholin glands or Skein's glands, not treatable by topical therapies. A trial of single 2 mg intravaginal metronidazole cream resulted in a 50 % cure rate compared to an 88 % cure rate with systemic therapy [28].

Use of metronidazole or tinidazole is associated with potential side effects, including a metallic taste, headache, and a 12 % incidence of nausea [29]. Ingestion of alcohol should be avoided for 24 h preceding and up to 72 h following drug administration. Prolonged therapies of these agents can potentiate the effects of warfarin and impact phenytoin and lithium levels [30].

For patients with metronidazole allergy, Pearlman et al. have reported successful use of an "incremental" protocol for desensitization used in two patients [31]. The first step is to verify an immediate hypersensitivity reaction by placing a small amount of MetroGel-Vaginal® gel on the skin and observing for the development of a wheal. If the patient has a demonstrated reaction, desensitizing therapy may be performed in a setting able to handle anaphylactic shock (generally a hospital). Patients should be pretreated with antihistamine or corticosteroids. They should be monitored with blood pressure, electrocardiogram, and continuous measurement of O2 saturation. A crash cart and intubation tray should be available with trained personnel ready. Metronidazole is given intravenously starting at a 5-μg dose and increasing increments every 15–20 min as outlined in Metronidazole Desensitization Protocol [20].

No routine test of cure is needed for patients who are treated unless the patient remains symptomatic. In this case, the most likely cause of symptoms is reinfection. Inquire about sexual exposures since treatment and their timing in relation to partner's treatments. Reinfections can be treated as initial infections. Routine doses of metronidazole may be subtherapeutic in patients taking drugs such as phenytoin, which increase hepatic microsomal enzyme activity.

Resistance to metronidazole is emerging. Current estimates are that 2.5–5 % of infections are resistant to recommended or alternative treatments [32]. Because clusters of patients with highly resistant *T. vaginalis* have not been reported, Pattman suggested that the mechanisms of metronidazole resistance are likely to be idiosyncratic and unstable [33]. In resistant infections, the patient and partner should be treated with a 7-day course of metronidazole 500 mg twice a day. Both should undergo immediate tests of cure following completion of treatment. If the infection persists, use metronidazole 500 mg orally 4 times a day for 3–5 days. Side effects and complication rates (including irreversible neurological problems) increase at doses greater than 3 g daily. It should be noted that there are seven cases reported in the literature of metronidazole-induced acute pancreatitis [34]. Various combinations of tinidazole orally and vaginally have been reported to be effective in the treatment of metronidazole-resistant trichomonal infections. Sobel reported an 89 % cure rate with 1 g orally 3 times a day combined with 500 mg per vagina 3 times a day for 14 days [25].

Some infections require culture and sensitivity testing to determine metronidazole dosing and the appropriate route of administration (oral or intravenous). Technical assistance and consultation are available at the Centers for Disease Control and Prevention (http://www.cdc.gov/std/).

Partner Notification and Reporting Requirements

Although *trichomonas* is not reportable disease, it is important to have partners treated before resuming sexual contract. If this does not take place, reinfection of the treated patient is almost a certainty. Caution patients that most men will deny any symptoms and may resist treatment, but they should be treated presumptively for *trichomonas* and related STIs even in the absence of any clinical finding of *T. vaginalis* infection.

Pregnancy-Related Issues

Pregnancy complications include an increased incidence of premature rupture of membranes and increased preterm delivery rates and low-birthweight infants [35]. Treatment with metronidazole (Pregnancy Category B) does not appear to reduce this prenatal morbidity. The safety of tinidazole in pregnancy has not been established. Pregnant women with symptomatic infections should be treated with metronidazole 2 mg orally all at once at any trimester. This therapy minimizes fetal exposure. Reports have found no teratogenicity associated with in utero exposure even if administered in the first trimester [36, 37]. Treatment of asymptomatic pregnant women is more controversial. Metronidazole has been associated with higher risk of preterm delivery in women with prior history of preterm delivery compared with untreated asymptomatic controls in one double-blinded, placebo-controlled trial [37]. However, treatment might reduce the spread of this STI and might prevent respiratory or genital infection of the newborn. The CDC does not recommend treatment of asymptomatic pregnant women. Breastfeeding women should discard their breast milk during treatment and for 12–24 h after their last dose of metronidazole. If using tinidazole, breast milk should be discarded for 3 days after the last dose.

Prevention

The National Institutes of Health expert panel cited a study that reports a 30 % reduction in risk of infection of *T. vaginalis* in women using condoms, but concludes that the paucity of epidemiological studies of condom effectiveness for *trichomonas* does not allow an accurate assessment of the reduction in risk of *trichomonas* infection by condom use [38].

Education regarding transmission of *T. vaginalis* and the signs and symptoms of trichomoniasis is needed by patients and providers. The health risks associated with trichomonal infection must be more respected, especially its connection with transmission of HIV. Health care professionals should adopt effective techniques for detection of this infection to reduce its prevalence. Patients need instruction in safer sex practices to avoid this infection.

Case Study

Angela, age 19, had a routine Pap smear, which indicated that she had an infection with *T. vaginalis*. Angela did not have a wet mount at the time of the Pap smear because she was asymptomatic. You treated her for *chlamydia* 4 months ago.

Questions

1. What should you do with the results?

Possible Answers

a. Perform a wet mount and treat only if the infection was confirmed.
b. Perform a wet mount and treat regardless of the outcome.
c. Culture her for *T. vaginalis*.
d. Decide that no follow-up is needed because she is asymptomatic.

Correct Answers

1 b. Try to find the infection on microscopy, but given that she is high risk, treat.

Teaching Points

- Sensitivity of the wet mount for detecting *trichomonas* is only 60 %; therefore, in an asymptomatic low-risk patient, confirmatory testing would be advisable.
- However, this patient, by virtue of her recent *chlamydia* diagnosis is a high-risk patient.
- Women and their partners need to be treated.
- A repeat *chlamydia* test should be done at the first visit. (It has been 4 months since her chlamydial cervicitis was treated.)
- A more comprehensive sexual history is indicated. This offers an opportunity for safer sex counseling.

References

1. Cates Jr W. Estimates of the incidence and prevalence of sexually transmitted diseases in the United States. American Social Health Association Panel. Sex Transm Dis. 1999;26:S2–7.
2. Gerbase AC, Rowley JT, Heymann DH, Berkley SF, Piot P. Global prevalence and incidence estimates of selected curable STDs. Sex Transm Infect. 1998;74:S12–6.
3. World Health Organization. Sexually Transmitted Infections Fact Sheet. Geneva, Switzerland: World Health Organization. 2004. Available from: www.who.int/reproductive-health/rtis/docs/sti_factsheet_2004.pdf. Accessed April 18, 2005.
4. Soper D. Trichomoniasis: under control or undercontrolled? Am J Obstet Gynecol. 2004;190:281–90.
5. Spence MR, Hollander DH, Smith J, McCaig L, Sewell D, Brockman M. The clinical and laboratory diagnosis of *Trichomonas vaginalis* infection. Sex Transm Dis. 1980;7:168–71.
6. Petrin D, Delgaty K, Bhatt R, Garber G. Clinical and microbiological aspects of *Trichomonas vaginalis*. Clin Microbiol Rev. 1998;11:300–17.
7. Horowitz BJ, Mårdh P-A, editors. Vaginitis and Vaginosis. New York, NY: Wiley-Liss; 1999.
8. Hook III EW. *Trichomonas vaginalis*—no longer a minor STD. Sex Transm Dis. 1999;26:388–9.
9. Laga M, Manoka A, Kivuvu M, et al. Non-ulcerative sexually transmitted diseases as risk factors for HIV-1 transmission in women: results from a cohort study. AIDS. 1993;7:95–102.
10. Hobbs MM, Kazembe P, Reed AW, et al. Trichomonas vaginalis as a cause of urethritis in Malawian men. Sex Transm Dis. 1999;26:381–7.
11. Thomason JL, Gelbart SM. Trichomonas vaginalis. Obstet Gynecol. 1989;74:536–41.
12. Latif AS, Mason PR, Marowa E. Urethral trichomoniasis in men. Sex Transm Dis. 1987;14:9–11.
13. Mason PR, Forman L. Serological survey of trichomoniasis in Zimbabwe Rhodesia. Cent Afr J Med. 1980;26:6–8.
14. Gardner HL, Dukes CD. Haemophilus vaginalis vaginitis: a newly defined specific infection previously classified non-specific vaginitis. Am J Obstet Gynecol. 1955;69:962–76.
15. Sweet RL, Gibbs RS. Infectious diseases of the female genital tract. 4th ed. Philadelphia, PA: Lippincott Williams & Wilkins; 2002. p. 339–40.
16. Lara-Torre E, Pinkerton JS. Accuracy of detection of *Trichomonas vaginalis* organisms on a liquid-based Papanicolaou smear. Am J Obstet Gynecol. 2003;188:354–6.

17. Ledger WJ, Monif GR. A growing concern: inability to diagnose vulvovaginal infections correctly. Obstet Gynecol. 2004;103:782–4.
18. Krieger JN, Tam MR, Stevens CE, et al. Diagnosis of trichomoniasis. Comparison of conventional wet-mount examination with cytologic studies, cultures, and monoclonal antibody staining of direct specimens. JAMA. 1988;259:1223–7.
19. van Der Schee C, van Belkum A, Zwijgers L, et al. Improved diagnosis of *Trichomonas vaginalis* infection by PCR using vaginal swabs and urine specimens compared to diagnosis by wet mount microscopy, culture, and fluorescent staining. J Clin Microbiol. 1999;37:4127–30.
20. Lobo TT, Feijo G, Carvalho SE, et al. A comparative evaluation of the Papanicolaou test for the diagnosis of trichomoniasis. Sex Transm Dis. 2003;30:694–9.
21. Borchardt KA, Li Z, Zhang MZ, Shing H. An in vitro metronidazole susceptibility test for trichomoniasis using the InPouch TV test. Genitourin Med. 1996;72:132–5.
22. Weston TE, Nicol CS. Natural history of trichomonal infection in males. Br J Vener Dis. 1963;39:251–7.
23. Durel P, Roiron V, Siboulet A, Borel LJ. Systemic treatment of human trichomoniasis with a derivative of nitro-imidazole, 8823 RP. Br J Vener Dis. 1960;36:21–6.
24. Centers for Disease Control and Prevention. Sexually transmitted diseases treatment guidelines, 2006. MMWR 2006; 55(RR-11):52–54. Available from: http://www.cdc.gov/std/treatment/. Accessed Nov. 24, 2006.
25. Sobel JD, Nyirjesy P, Brown W. Tinidazole therapy for metronidazole-resistant vaginal trichomoniasis. Clin Infect Dis. 2001;33:1341–6.
26. Spence MR, Harwell TS, Davies MC, Smith JL. The minimum single oral metronidazole dose for treating trichomoniasis: a randomized, blinded study. Obstet Gynecol. 1997;89:699–703.
27. Hager WD, Brown ST, Kraus SJ, Kleris GS, Perkins GJ, Henderson M. Metronidazole for vaginal trichomoniasis. Seven-day vs single-dose regimens. JAMA. 1980;244:1219–20.
28. Tidwell BH, Lushbaugh WB, Laughlin MD, Cleary JD, Finley RW. A double-blind placebo-controlled trial of single-dose intravaginal versus single-dose oral metronidazole in the treatment of trichomonal vaginitis. J Infect Dis. 1994;170:242–6.
29. Smilack JD, Wilson WR, Cockerill III FR. Tetracyclines, chloramphenicol, erythromycin, clindamycin, and metronidazole. Mayo Clin Proc. 1991;66:1270–80.
30. Flagyl. Prescribing Information. Chicago, IL: Pfizer Inc., 2004.
31. Pearlman MD, Yashar C, Ernst S, Solomon W. An incremental dosing protocol for women with severe vaginal trichomoniasis and adverse reaction to metronidazole. Am J Obstet Gynecol. 1996;174:934–6.
32. Schmid G, Narcisi E, Mosure D, Secor WE, Higgins J, Moreno H. Prevalence of metronidazole-resistant *Trichomonas vaginalis* in a gynecology clinic. J Reprod Med. 2001;46:545–9.
33. Pattman RS. Recalcitrant vaginal trichomoniasis. Sex Transm Infect. 1999;75:127–8.
34. Feola DJ, Thornton AC. Metronidazole-induced pancreatitis in a patient with recurrent vaginal trichomoniasis. Pharmacotherapy. 2002;22:1508–10.
35. Cotch MF, Pastorek II JG, Nugent RP, et al. *Trichomonas vaginalis* associated with low birth weight and preterm delivery. The Vaginal Infections and Prematurity Study Group. Sex Transm Dis. 1997;24:353–60.
36. Burtin P, Taddio A, Ariburnu O, Einarson TR, Koren G. Safety of metronidazole in pregnancy: a meta-analysis. Am J Obstet Gynecol. 1995;172:525–9.
37. Piper JM, Mitchel EF, Ray WA. Prenatal use of metronidazole and birth defects: no association. Obstet Gynecol. 1993;82:348–52.
38. National Institute of Allergy and Infectious Diseases. Workshop summary: scientific evidence on condom effectiveness for sexually transmitted disease (STD) prevention. Washington, DC: National Institutes of Health, Department of Health Services, 2001. Available from: http://www.niaid.nih.gov/dmid/stds/condomreport.pdf. Accessed Nov. 24, 2006.

Chapter 10
Lymphogranuloma Venereum, Chancroid, Granuloma Inguinale, and Molluscum Contagiosum

Jo Ann Woodward

Introduction

Genital infections with lymphogranuloma venereum (LGV), chancroid, granuloma inguinale, and molluscum contagiosum are sexually transmitted infections (STIs) that are generally more frequently found in tropical areas, but do present in the United States. Each is more common in human immunodeficiency virus (HIV)-infected individuals than in the general population. Ulcerative infections increase the risks of transmission and acquisition of HIV. Diagnosis of each of these infections is usually done clinically; the availability of laboratory testing to support the diagnosis is limited.

Fast Facts

- Chancroid lesions are very painful and often spread by auto-inoculation, especially in women.
- LGV initially presents as a painless lesion that may go unnoticed, but the subsequent adenopathy can be very painful. In the third stage of the disease, fibrosis causes significant genital distortion, including elephantiasis.
- Granuloma inguinale is also a chronic, ulcerative, progressively destructive STI. In the advanced stages, the lesions swell, become superinfected, and induce irreversible genital deformity. Social isolation is common because of the characteristic aroma of this infection.
- Molluscum contagiosum in the genital area is an STI. The characteristic lesion is a raised, centrally umbilicated papule or nodule.

J.A. Woodward, WHNP-BC (✉)
Scottsdale, AZ 85258, USA
e-mail: npjoann@aol.com

N.S. Skolnik et al. (eds.), *Sexually Transmitted Diseases: A Practical Guide for Primary Care*, Current Clinical Practice, DOI 10.1007/978-1-62703-499-9_10, © Springer Science+Business Media New York 2013

Lymphogranuloma Venereum

Introduction

LGV was not identified as a separate pathological entity until 1913. Before that time, it was confused with chancroid, syphilis, or herpes. It has also been called tropical, strumous, climatic bubo, lymphogranuloma inguinale, poradenitis inguinalis, and Durand–Nicolas–Favre disease [1]. LGV is a chronic STI caused by *Chlamydia trachomatis*. LGV has three stages of clinical manifestations—a small, short-lived, relatively asymptomatic primary lesion; a secondary stage characterized by inguinal adenopathy or acute hemorrhagic proctitis and systemic symptoms; and a third stage marked by ulceration, fistula formation, rectal strictures, and genital elephantiasis. Because of the ulcerative nature of LGV, patients are at increased risk of transmitting or acquiring HIV and other STIs.

Prevalence and Incidence

Although LGV is found worldwide, it most commonly occurs in tropical areas. LGV is endemic in East and West Africa, India, part of Southeast Asia, Central American, South American, and the Caribbean. For example, a surveyed clinic in Ethiopia reported several thousand cases each year [1]. By contrast, LGV is relatively rare in the United States and occurs sporadically. In 2004, there was a slight increase in cases reported among men who have sex with men (MSM) on the west coast. Most cases in the United States are found in men and in urban areas. Peak years of infection are in the 30s. Although LGV infections are 5 times more likely to occur in men than in women, the long-term complications are more common in women because the infection is more asymptomatic in women and, therefore, more frequently goes undetected until a more advanced stage.

Risk Factors

As an STI, the risk of the infection is increased by a history of multiple sexual partners and young age. However, in the most recent outbreaks in the United States, most cases were found among MSM practicing anal-receptive sex who have had contact with MSM from Europe. Travel to endemic countries is another risk factor in those engaging in high-risk sexual practices.

Infectivity and Transmission

LGV is spread by sexual contact. It is not known if LGV can be transmitted as a fomite on shared sex toys or by fisting, which would be important to know when counseling MSM [2]. The infectivity is not known, but is generally thought to be less than gonorrhea.

Etiology

LGV is an STI caused by *C. trachomatis*, serotypes L1, L2, and L3. *C. trachomatis* cannot penetrate intact skin or mucous membranes. It enters the body through micro-abrasions in the skin. The life cycle of *C. trachomatis* is discussed in Chap. 5. These strains are more invasive in tissue culture than the strains that cause chlamydial cervi-citis and urethritis. It is believed that most of the extensive tissue damage seen with LGV is caused by a cell-mediated "hypersensitivity" to chlamydia antigen [3].

Clinical Manifestation

The incubation period for LGV is 3–30 days. The disease has both systemic mani-festations and a wide spectrum of anogenital lesions, lymphadenopathy with destruction, and distortion of the genital areas. Subclinical infections are also pos-sible, especially in women. The clinical manifestations progress through three stages. The primary lesion is generally self-limited and painless except in primary rectal LGV, which may present with proctitis and diarrhea, discharge, and ulcer-ations [4]. The primary lesion, which develops at the site of inoculation, is typically small (2–10 mm in diameter). This primary lesion can take one of four forms: a small, nonpainful papule; a shallow ulcer or erosion; a small herpetiform lesion; or nonspecific urethritis [1]. The primary lesion usually bursts quickly and forms an ulcer that oozes pus, but heals rapidly thereafter. In women, the lesion typically forms in the posterior vaginal wall, the fourchette, cervix, or vulva. In men, the primary lesion occurs in the coronal sulcus, but may develop on the frenulum, pre-puce, penis, urethral glans, or scrotum. It may be associated with a cordlike lym-phangitis of the dorsal penis and form large painful lymphangial nodule called a "bubonulus" [1]. If the bubonulus ruptures, both draining sinuses of the urethra and deforming scars on the penis can develop. In women, LGV cervicitis can spread into the parametrium or salpinges. Alternatively, the lesion may remain undetected in the urethra, vaginal vault, or rectum as it ulcerates.

Most people first seek care during the second stage of the infection because the first stage goes unnoticed by them. The secondary stage of LGV represents the spread of the infection into lymphatic tissue. The secondary stage develops days to months (average 10–30 days) after the primary lesion. The first symptoms of the second stage may be systemic—such as fever, malaise, headache, anorexia, myalgia, and arthralgia. In the inguinal syndrome, these symptoms are followed rapidly by the development of adenopathy. The inguinal syndrome is the most frequent clinical manifestation of LGV. The superficial inguinal nodes are most often involved, but femoral nodes may also be affected. Adenopathy is unilateral in two-thirds of cases in women. Initially firm, discrete, multiple, slightly tender nodes develop. As the inflammation of the lymph nodes becomes more intense in the following few weeks, the nodes enlarge, necrose, and form fluctuant abscesses or buboes. These become adherent to the subcutaneous tissue and the overlying skin. If both the inguinal and femoral nodes are involved, Poupart's ligament creates a groove between the nodes and the patient develops the classic "groove sign"; this occurs in 10–20 % of cases [3]. If untreated, the bubo ruptures in one-third of cases. Rupture relieves the pain and fever, but multiple sinus tracts form in the base of the ulcer and drain thick pus for months. Even after rupture, buboes recur in 20 % of untreated patients [1]. Buboes that do not rupture undergo slow involution and form chronic inguinal masses.

Another second stage manifestation of LGV is the anogenitorectal syndrome, in which perianal or perirectal lymphatic tissue (usually of the distal left side of the large intestine) becomes inflamed, resulting in hemorrhagic proctocolitis, perirectal abscesses, ischiorectal or rectovaginal fistulas, or anal fistulas. Ultimately, anal or rectal strictures result. The clinical and histological presentations of LGV proctocolitis may mimic the initial manifestations of inflammatory bowel disease [5]. The rectal strictures of LGV must be distinguished from carcinoma, tuberculosis, actinomycosis, and schistosomiasis.

A minority of patients infected with LGV will progress to the third stage of the infection, which involves the external genitalia and the rectal area. Because healing from LGV infection is by fibrosis, the normal structure of the lymph nodes is altered, which causes obstruction of the lymphatics of the scrotum, penis, or vulva. The chronic infection of the lymphatics, and the resulting edema and sclerosing fibrosis of the subcutaneous tissue cause induration and enlargement. This presents clinically as elephantiasis. In men, elephantiasis occurs within the penoscrotal area.

It is believed that much of the tissue damage in LGV is caused by a cell-mediated hypersensitivity to chlamydia antigens [3]. The term esthiomene, which is derived from the Greek word for "eating away," is used to describe the findings of LGV of the lymphatic system of the vulva, penis, and scrotum [1]. Ulceration of the lesion starts superficially, but later becomes destructive. In women, the areas of the labia major, genitocrural folds, and lateral areas of the perineum are most frequently involved.

Other clinical presentations include papillary growths in the urethral meatus of women, smooth pedunculated perianal lesions ("lymphorrhoids"), and follicular conjunctivitis. Rarely, the infecting organism enters the blood stream and involves unusual sites, such as the gallbladder, liver, or pericardium. Primary infections of the oral cavity or pharynx have also been reported.

Diagnosis

Diagnosis is based primarily on clinical findings; routine laboratory confirmation may not be possible [6]. However, given the wide variety of clinical manifestations, clinical diagnosis may be difficult. This difficulty is compounded by the relative rarity of this infection, which means that many clinicians may not recognize the clinical findings.

Serological tests such as microimmunofluorescent or complement fixation tests are most commonly used to support the clinical diagnosis. Titers of complement fixation tests more than 1:64, or a fourfold increase in titer, are considered diagnostic [3] as are titers more than 1:128 on the microimmunofluorescent test [7]. A list of laboratories that perform serologic tests for *C. trachomatis* and might provide titered results is available from http://www.cdc.gov/std/lgv-labs.htm.

The most accurate tests used to diagnose LGV today are those using polymerase chain reaction (PCR) and other amplification techniques, although non-culture nucleic acid testing is not specific for LGV. The Food and Drug Administration has not approved the use of rectal swabs for nucleic acid testing [6]. In research settings and specialized laboratories, the genotype can be determined by performing restriction endonuclease pattern analysis of the amplified outer membrane protein A gene. Cultures of aspirates from the buboes or lesions are often performed, but are positive in only 30–50 % of suspected lesions [1, 8].

Evaluation of gastrointestinal syndromes that may have been sexually transmitted requires either anoscopy or sigmoidoscopy and testing for *C. trachomatis*, syphilis, herpes, *N. gonorrhoeae*, and common enteric pathogens that can be sexually transmitted [6]. In order to evaluate rectal strictures, mucosal biopsy may be needed to rule out carcinoma or other chronic infections.

Treatment

The treatment of LGV is displayed in Table 10.1. Treatment should be started empirically pending return of laboratory test results. If the laboratory test results all return negative, therapy can be discontinued, if appropriate. The goal is to cure the infection and prevent ongoing tissue damage. Antibiotics are needed for 3 weeks. In addition, buboes may require aspiration through intact, uninfected tissue or incision and drainage to prevent inguinal/femoral ulcerations. Patients should be followed clinically until all signs and symptoms have resolved.

Table 10.1 Lymphogranuloma venereum CDC STD treatment guidelines 2010

Recommended regimen	Alternative regimen
Doxycycline[a]	Erythromycin base[b]
100 mg orally twice a day for 21 days	500 mg orally 4 times a day for 21 days

Source: Ref [6]

[a]Contraindicated for pregnant and lactating women and for children under 8 years old

Partner Notification and Reporting Requirements

All partners who have had sexual contact with the patient within 60 days of the onset of symptoms should be examined [6, 7]. In the absence of symptoms, sexual contacts should be treated for a chlamydia cervicitis or urethritis (see Table 5.3 in Chap. 5). Symptomatic partners should be treated according to LGV treatment guidelines outlined in Table 10.1. If the patient is in the second stage of the infection, earlier partners may benefit from therapy. LGV is a reportable infection in many large metropolitan cities (Los Angeles, New York, and so on), but case reporting is not mandatory in all public health jurisdictions [9].

Pregnancy-Related Issues

Transplacental congenital infection can occur, but most neonatal infection occurs because of exposure during passage through an infected birth canal. For infected pregnant and lactating women, the Centers for Disease Control and Prevention (CDC) recommends only the use of erythromycins. Doxycycline is contraindicated in pregnancy.

Chancroid

Introduction

Chancroid is commonly referred to as "soft chancre." It is a highly contagious STI caused by *Haemophilus ducreyi*. *H. ducreyi* was first identified as the causative organism for chancroid in 1889 when August Ducrey inoculated the forearms of infected patients with pus from their genital lesions [10]. Causation was made even clearer later when Bezancon et al. inoculated the forearms of healthy volunteers with culture-purified organisms (*H. ducreyi*) and produced characteristic soft chancres from which the organisms were re-isolated [11].

The infection causes genital ulceration, regional lymphatitis, and bubo formation. It is a major cause of genital ulcer disease in many resource-poor countries in Africa, Asia, and Latin America [12]. The genital ulceration caused by chancroid causes significant distress and increases the transmission and acquisition of HIV infection [13]. The relative risk of acquiring HIV if a genital ulcer is present ranges from 3 to 18, with a per act increase in transmission of 10- to 100-fold [14]. About 10 % of the US patients with chancroids are co-infected with HIV or *Treponema pallidum*; this rate is higher than the rate found in infected individuals in other countries.

Prevalence/Incidence

In 1997, the World Health Organization estimated that six million cases of chancroid occurred worldwide each year [15]. In developing countries, chancroid is the cause of most genital ulcerative disease and accounts for 10–30 % of all STIs in Africa. In tropical countries, such as Kenya and Thailand, chancroid is one of the most common STIs [16]. The infection is common in Africa, Southeast Asia, and the Caribbean [17]. In developed countries, chancroid occurs sporadically, and most frequently among those individuals who have traveled to endemic areas. In the United States, 80 % of infections occur in heterosexual men. The male-to-female ratio of infection in the United States is between 5:1 and 10:1.

Risk Factors

Commercial sex workers are felt to have been reservoirs of infection in the outbreaks that have occurred in the United States in the last decade. This is because chancroid is most commonly diagnosed in men who have recent exposure. Uncircumcised men are more susceptible to infection [18].

Infectivity and Transmissibility

Chancroid is a relatively contagious infection. Estimates are that 70 % of women who are sex partners of chancroid-infected men are infected [19]. The probability of sexual transmission with a single exposure has been estimated to be 0.35 [20]. An estimated delivery dose of approximately 30 colony-forming units of *H. ducreyi* organisms has been reported to form a papule formation rate of 95 % and a pustule formation rate of 69 % in a human experimental challenge model [21].

Etiology

Chancroid is caused by a small, nonmobile facultative anaerobic, Gram-negative rod bacterium, *H. ducreyi*. The organism is only remotely related to Haemophilus influenza and has been reclassified in the *Actinobacillus* cluster of the Pasteurellae [14]. *H. ducreyi* only infects humans. It is believed that the organism gains entry into the skin and mucosal surfaces only through microabrasions and other trauma; it is not able to penetrate normal skin.

Clinical Manifestations

The lesions of chancroid are generally limited to the genital areas. In women, they are found on the labia, clitoris, vestibule, and fourchette. In men, the lesions are most commonly cited in the inner surface of the prepuce and frenulum.

The incubation period of chancroid is 3–11 days, with the most common frequency being 4–7 days. A small papule develops at the site of entry. The papule is haloed by erythema. In 2–3 days, the lesion becomes pustular or vesiculopustular, and ulcerates. The base of the ulcer is soft, shallow, and necrotic-appearing; the edges are irregular, ragged, and undermined and are surrounded by deep red-colored halos. The ulcers are covered by a grey-colored, foul-smelling exudate. There is no induration around the lesion. The lesion is exquisitely painful and tender. In men, the most common initial presentation is a single ulcer. In women, multiple ulcers form and often become interconnected in serpentine streaks measuring up to 2 cm. Many times, they are bilateral (the so-called kissing lesions) created by auto-inoculation. Mixed infections with syphilis and herpes simplex can complicate the diagnosis of chancroid.

In 7–10 days, a bubo develops in about half the cases. The bubo is unilateral (same side as lesion) and unilocular in up to two-thirds of the time. It is an acute, painful, tender inflammatory inguinal adenopathy. Untreated buboes may rupture and form large weeping ulcers in the inguinal area. Phimosis may develop in men. Extragenital infections are possible but rare.

Symptoms in men relate to the lesions themselves; the pain of the lesion of the adenopathy will prompt men to seek professional care. In women, the symptoms generally are more nonspecific; infected women complain of dysuria, dyspareunia, vaginal discharge, or rectal bleeding depending on the location of infection.

Relapses after antibiotic therapy occur in up to 5 % of patients.

Diagnostic Testing

The classical presentation of a painful ulcer and tender suppurative inguinal adenopathy is almost pathognomonic for chancroid. However, this complex occurs in only about one-third of cases. Therefore, the diagnosis of chancroid generally relies on other tests. The exudates from the lesion or from aspiration of the lesion may reveal the Gram-negative rods extracellularly located in chains with clustering. The Gram stain patterns of *H. ducreyi* have been described as "schools of fish," "railroad tracks," and "fingerprints." However, the sensitivity of the Gram stain is only 50 %, and should not be used to rule out chancroid [22]. Definitive laboratory diagnosis depends on culture and isolation of *H. ducreyi*; but those tests are rarely available in standard labs. Even in the best of situations, the sensitivity of cultures is only about 80 %. Because *H. ducreyi* is so fastidious, it must be plated directly onto the culture media or plated on Stuart's, Amies', and thioglycolate hemin-based transport media and transported at 4 °C.

PCR and multiplex PCR tests have been described for *H. ducreyi*, but none has received Food and Drug Administration approval. The PCR tests lose sensitivity when used to test genital ulcer specimens but are still superior to culture tests [12]. Multiplex PCR is particularly useful in the face of coinfection, because it can detect the presence of *H. ducreyi* as well as herpes simplex virus, and *T. pallidum* [23].

Studies have shown that the accuracy of clinical diagnosis of *H. ducreyi* infection is related to the prevalence of chancroid in the population, as well as the experience of the clinician [12]. Overall, the accuracy ranges from 33 to 80 % [24, 25]. Also complicating this situation is the fact that coinfection of HIV and *H. ducreyi* is common. HIV can modify the appearance of chancroid [12].

Despite these limitations, the diagnosis is often made on clinical grounds, and testing is used to rule out other infections that cause genital ulceration, such as syphilis or herpes. The CDC recommends that the probable diagnosis of chancroid be made if:

- The individual has one or more painful genital ulcers.
- There is no evidence of syphilis by dark-field examination of the lesions, or by serology performed at least 7 days after the onset of the ulcers.
- Either the clinical presentation of the genital ulcers and regional adenopathy are typical for chancroid or test results for herpes simplex virus are negative.

Patients diagnosed with chancroid should be tested for HIV, not only because of the high concordance but also because HIV-infected patients do not respond to therapy as well.

Treatment

The CDC treatment guidelines are for chancroid outlined. The agents currently used are more expensive than the traditional treatments based on tetracycline or penicillin. Resistance to chloramiphene, sulfonamide, and amino-glycosides has emerged [26]. Azithromycin and ceftriaxone have the advantage of being single-dose therapies.

Patients should be reexamined within 3–7 days of initiation of therapy. If treatment is successful, the patient should improve symptomatically within 3 days. The clinical appearance should improve within 7 days. If the patient does not improve adequately within 7 days, there are several possibilities:

- The diagnosis was incorrect.
- The diagnosis was incomplete and the patient was co-infected with another STI.
- The strain of *H. ducreyi* is resistant to the antibiotic given.
- The treatment was not correctly taken.
- The patient is immunocompromised, as with HIV infection.

The time to complete healing depends on the size of the ulcer. Larger ulcers may require more than 14 days to heal. Ulcers located under the foreskin of uncircumcised men are also slower to heal; uncircumcised men also have higher treatment failure rates.

The bubo (fluctuant adenopathy) may require aspiration through uninfected adjacent tissue. Buboes larger than 5 cm may need incision and drainage. After aspiration, fluid may re-accumulate; repeated aspirations may be required until healing is complete.

HIV-infected patients require closer and more prolonged monitoring because they are more likely to respond slowly or inadequately to conventional therapy. They may also require longer courses of antibiotics.

In developing countries with little or no ability to perform diagnostic testing, the World Health Organization recommends the use of a symptomatic management approach for genital ulcer disease. Symptomatic management calls for patients to be treated at the first visit with a combination of antibiotics that treat the sexually transmitted diseases (STDs) commonly found locally [27]. This means that neither clinical experience nor laboratory support is needed. It has been shown to be more successful that traditional targeted and therapies in management of genital ulcers in Rwanda [28].

Patients should avoid sexual contact until the ulcers are completely healed.

Partner Notification and Reporting Requirements

Sex partners of patients who had contact with the infected patient in the 10 days preceding the onset of the patient's symptoms should be examined. Treatment should be given even if the contact is asymptomatic. Chancroid is a reportable disease.

Pregnancy-Related Issues

No direct adverse effects of chancroid infection have been demonstrated on the pregnancy or on the neonate. Ciprofloxacin is contraindicated in pregnancy and lactation. The CDC 2006 guidelines also state that the safety and efficacy of azithromycin for pregnant or lactating women have not been established and recommend in favor of other agents. However, other expert panels have not limited the use of azithromycin in those patients [29].

Granuloma Inguinale

Introduction

Granuloma inguinale, also known as Donovanosis, is a chronic, ulcerative, progressively destructive bacterial infection of the genital and anal skin and subcutaneous tissue caused by the bacterium *Klebsiella granulomatis* (formerly known as Calymmatobacterium granulomatis). It is classified as an STI because it is spread predominantly by sexual contact, but it can be spread by other means.

The differential includes other causes of genital ulceration (syphilis, LGV, herpes, chancroid), other granulomatous conditions, and carcinomas. When a biopsy from a large necrotic lesion that appears neoplastic shows only inflammatory changes, consider granuloma inguinale and order special stains to reveal K. granulomatis.

Prevalence/Incidence

This infection rarely occurs in the United States but granuloma inguinale is endemic in some tropical and developing areas, including India, southern Africa, Papua New Guinea, central Australia, and the Caribbean islands. In the United States, fewer than 100 cases are reported each year. Infection is more common in men; the male-to-female ratio is about 2.5:1 [30]. Infection rates peak among 20- to 30-year olds.

Infectivity/Transmissibility

The infection can be spread as an STI, but can also be spread by close, personal, nonsexual contact. It is not highly contagious; usually repeated or chronic exposure is needed to contract the infection. The infection is found in 1–52 % of sexual partners of women with the infection [31]. It is also found in sexually abstinent children and very old adults without sexual contact, which suggests that nonsexual transmission is possible. Indirect contact through vaginal contamination by fecal organisms may be an important contributor, as auto-inoculation may be [30].

Etiology

Granuloma inguinale is caused by an intracellular Gram-negative bacterium K. granulomatis. This organism is a small (0.1 µm), nonmotile, non-sporing, encapsulated coccobacillus that shares common antigens with *Klebsiella* and *Escherichia coli.* It may be part of the intestinal flora, which is made pathogenic by a bacterio-phage [30]. *K. granulomatous* is pathogenic only for humans and chick embryos.

Clinical Presentation

Granuloma inguinale is an acute or chronic infection characterized by ulcerating, nec-rosing, superinfected lesions of the skin, and subcutaneous tissues in the anogenital area. The incubation period varies from 1 to 2 weeks. The initial lesion of granuloma inguinale can be single or multiple papules. In women, the usual sites of infection are the inner aspect of labia and fourchette. In men, the lesions are generally found on the penis. In 10 % of cases, the initial lesion develops in the inguinal area. The lesion is friable and bleeds easily on contact. The skin over each nodule ulcerates. The charac-teristic lesion is an area of coalesced beefy-red ulcers with fresh granular tissue. As the adjacent areas of ulceration grow together, the normal vulvar/penile architecture is destroyed. The lesion is generally not painful and there is minimal adenopathy. Four different types of granuloma inguinale have been described [32]:

- Ulcerogranulomatosis (the most common type) marked by beefy-red, non-tender ulcers that bleed easily if touched and may become quite extensive if not treated.
- Hypertrophic or verrucous ulcer, which presents as a growth with an irregular edge.
- Necrotic type with a foul-smelling, deep ulcer causing tissue destruction.
- Dry, sclerotic, or cicatricial lesion.

Massive swelling of the labia is common. Inguinal swelling may occur, but not because of enlarged or obstructed lymph nodes. Instead, "pseudo buboes" form because of subcutaneous granulation. The pseudo buboes break down and are replaced by ulcers. Adenopathy may develop in response to bacterial infection of the ulcerated lesions. Social isolation is common because of the smell of the infected tissue.

As the infection progresses, scarring and lymphatic obstruction produce marked enlargement of the vulvar area. Although correct treatment can eradicate the infec-tion, long-standing infection can cause irreversible genital deformities such as skin depigmentation; stenosis of the urethral, vaginal, and anal orifices; and massive edema [30]. Loss of sexual function often follows because of destruction of genital tissue, scarring, and deformities [33].

Relapse of granuloma inguinale is relatively frequent and may occur 6–18 months after apparently effective treatment [34].

Extragenital lesions have been reported up to 6 % of cases. Involvement on the face, neck, mouth, larynx, pharynx, and chest have all been reported. Metastatic lesions involving bones, joints, and liver have been reported [30]. The patients affected with these distant lesions often had cervical or uterine disease.

Diagnosis

In endemic areas, the infection is usually diagnosed by its clinical presentation. Identification of Donovan bodies using special stains in either smears or crushed specimens taken from the depth of the ulcer and the fresh edge confirms the clinical diagnosis. Biopsies should be taken with punch biopsy or small curettes. Air-dry the specimen then fix in 95 % ethanol for 5 min. The specimen should then be stained. Donovan bodies are seen on Giemsa stain or Wright stain as clusters of dark-staining bacteria that appear as small, straight, or curved dumbbell-shaped "safety pin" (bipolar) appearance in the cytoplasm of macrophages. They stain purple with a surrounding pink capsule. In patients who have taken even small amounts of small antibiotics, however, the Donovan bodies may not be present. Biopsy may be necessary to rule out carcinoma.

Standard laboratory approaches are not fruitful. *K. granulomatosis* is difficult to culture; it has been cultured successfully only in chick embryonic yoke sac [35]. A PCR test has been developed using swabs rather than biopsy or tissue samples, but this is not readily available [36, 37]. In vitro antibiotic sensitivity testing is unavailable [38]. Serological tests are nonspecific.

Treatment

The granuloma inguinale treatment guidelines recommended by the CDC are outlined in Table 10.2. In general, at least 3 weeks of broad-spectrum antibiotics are necessary. Therapy should be continued until there is healing of all ulcers. This requires prolonged self-administration, which raises the possibility of poor compliance. Poor compliance increases the likelihood of antibiotic resistance, reducing the observed cure rates, and raising community and patient dissatisfaction. This in turn increases the likelihood of poor compliance [33].

Initial response should be recognizable within 7 days, although maximal effect may take 3–5 weeks to see. Tetracycline resistance is widespread. Gentamicin should be added if the lesions fail to respond after the first few days of therapy. The advanced lesions seen in endemic areas respond poorly to conventional treatment regimens.

Partner Notification and Reporting Requirements

Individuals who had sexual contact with a patient in the 60 days before the onset of the patient's symptoms should be contacted and offered testing. Empiric therapy in asymptomatic partners has not been studied, but given the low infectivity of this organism, it is not recommended at this time. Reporting to the local health departments is necessary.

Table 10.2 Granuloma inguinale (donovanosis) CDC STD treatment guidelines 2010

Recommended regimen		Alternative regimens	Select one of the following
Doxycycline a	100 mg orally twice a day for at least 3 weeks	Azithromycin	1 g orally once per week for at least 3 weeks
		Ciprofloxacin c	750 mg orally twice a day for at least 3 weeks
		Erythromycin base	500 mg orally 4 times a day for at least 3 weeks
		Trimethoprim	One double-strength tablet
		Sulfamethoxazole b	One (800 mg/160 mg) tablet orally twice a day for at least 3 weeks

Source: ref. [6].

CDC Centers for Disease Control and Prevention; *STD* sexually transmitted disease

Therapy should be continued at least 3 weeks or until all lesions have completely healed. Some specialists recommend the addition of an aminoglycoside to the above regimens if improvement is not evident within the first few days of therapy (e.g., Gentamicin, 1 mg/kg IV every 8 h)

a Contraindicated for pregnant and lactating women and for children under 8 years old

b Pregnancy is a relative contraindication to the use of sulfonamides

c Contraindicated for pregnant and lactating women

Pregnancy-Related Issues

There have been no reports of congenital transmission of this infection, but transmission may occur during vaginal delivery. Otitis media and mastoiditis have been reported in exposed children, so careful cleansing of the heads of newborns born to infected mothers is recommended [39]. In pregnancy, women tend to have less genital tract bleeding and fewer sites of infection. Erythromycin is the recommended treatment agent, but the addition of gentamicin is highly advisable. Azithromycin might prove useful for treating a granuloma in pregnancy, but data is lacking.

Molluscum Contagiosum

Introduction

Molluscum contagiosum is a viral infection that is an increasingly common prevalence, especially in those infected with HIV. The characteristic lesion is a raised, umbilicated papule or nodule. The lesions are self-limited, but may persist for up to 5 years. Molluscum is often sexually transmitted in adults, but it may be asexually transmitted in children.

Prevalence/Incidence

Molluscum contagiosum is found worldwide, but has higher prevalence in tropical areas. Its incidence is estimated to be between 2 and 8 % [40]. Statistics in the United States are not available; indirect evidence suggests that it is increasing in frequency of diagnosis. Molluscum contagiosum accounts for 1 % of all diagnosed dermatological conditions [41]. In the last 30 years, the number of molluscum-related office visits increased dramatically [42]. The infection is most frequently found in patients in the 15- to 29-year-old age range. Estimates are that 5–18 % of HIV-infected patients are also infected with molluscum contagiosum [43]. The disease is endemic with a higher incidence within institutions and communities where overcrowding, poor hygiene, and poverty enable its spread [42].

Infectivity/Transmissibility

The virus is spread by direct skin contact with an infected individual, and is often spread sexually in adolescents and adults. It develops more frequently in patients who have deficient cell-mediated immunity. The communicability of molluscum contagiosum is not known, but the condition is known to be only mildly contagious [44]. Transmission of the virus is also possible by fomites (e.g., bath towels, tattooing instruments, equipment in beauty parlors and Turkish baths, as well as underwear) as well as by auto-inoculation [42].

Etiology

Molluscum contagiosum is a member of the pox virus (Poxviridae) family, to which small pox and variola also belong. Pox viruses are complex, double-stranded DNA viruses that contain an envelope. The virus infects only squamous skin, not mucous membranes.

Pox viruses enter cells by endocytosis or by cell fusion. They then uncoat, and transcription of the viral DNA takes place to produce infective virions. These intracytoplasmic virions can be seen microscopically. Intact virus is shed through the epidermis and spread over the skin. Infection with the virus causes hyperplasia and hypertrophy of the epidermis [45]. The molluscum bodies contain large numbers of maturing virions within a collagen-lipid-rich sac-like structure that evades host immunological detection [46].

Clinical Presentations

Incubation time averages 14–50 days [47], but can be as long as 6 months. Infections are usually self-limited, but can persist for up to 5 years [44]. Molluscum contagiosum causes lesions in adults and adolescents in the groin, genitalia, and lower abdomen. Younger children may develop asexually transmitted lesions on the face, truck, extremities, axilla, and crural folds. The lesions are generally discrete, smooth, firm, skin-colored (opalescent), raised (domed) lesions with central umbilication. "Water wart" is a descriptive term for the lesion. The central depression contains a white, waxy, or curd-like core. The lesions are either papules measuring 1–5 mm in diameter or larger nodules measuring 6–10 mm in diameter. They may appear as solitary lesions or clusters generally of less than 30 lesions.

Infections rarely cause inflammatory changes. However, trauma may rupture the lesions and cause acute inflammation [48]. Deep infections may have one or more shallow cysts filled with molluscum bodies.

The lesions are generally asymptomatic but may cause pruritus or tenderness. Lesions spread by sexual contact may appear in the perianal or perioral areas. In some cases, there may be eczema around the lesion, which resolves after the resolution of the lesion [44]. Bacterial superinfection of the lesion is a concern [31]. The appearance of the infection in immunocompromised patients may be atypical. HIV-infected patients also tend to grow giant lesions (>1 cm) or may have clusters of hundreds of small lesions. These lesions last longer and tend to spread to other locations (especially the face) and are more resistant to common treatments [44]. For the smaller lesions, the differential diagnosis includes condyloma acuminata or vulvar syringoma. For the larger, solitary lesions, carcinoma must be ruled out.

Diagnosis

Diagnosis of genital molluscum contagiosum is generally made based on the clinical appearance of the lesions. If there is any question, biopsy of the lesion with Gram, Wright, or Giemsa staining can be helpful. The most common histological feature of molluscum contagiosum is the intracytoplasmic purplish-to-red inclusion known as the molluscum body (Henderson-Patterson body) [49].

The virus cannot be grown in culture other than human skin as its host. On the vulva, molluscum contagiosum can coexist with condyloma acuminata, which can make identification of the lesions more challenging.

Treatment

A debate remains over the need to treat molluscum contagiosum, because it is a self-limited infection in most cases. Many clinicians recommend therapy to reduce the risk of transmission to sex partners and auto-inoculation, and for quality-of-life reasons [44].

Physician-administered ablative procedures are commonly used to treat molluscum. Cryotherapy is one of the most common, quick, and efficient methods oftreatment. Liquid nitrogen, dry ice, or Frigiderm may be applied to each lesion for a few seconds. Repeat treatments may be needed in 2- to 3-week intervals [50]. Hyperpigmentation, hypopigmentation, or scarring may be created by this treatment.

Enucleation of the molluscum body by needle or by curettage is also commonly used. The area is cleansed with an antiseptic agent, and the core of each lesion is removed. Silver nitrate, ferric subsulfate, or 85 % trichloroacetic acid is applied to the center for hemostasis. General curettage of the area to unroof lesions with a sharp dermal curette is more practical when there are numerous lesions present. Pulsed dye laser has also demonstrated excellent results in single treatment without scarring or pigment abnormalities [51]. Cost makes this approach less desirable [52]. Cantharidin (0.9 % solution of collodion and acetone) has been used with success in the treatment of molluscum contagiosum. This is a blister-inducing agent. It should be carefully applied to the dome of the lesion and left in place for 4 h before being washed off. If tolerated on a single test lesion, it may be applied to other lesions every week until clearance occurs. It should not be used on the face [53]. Use of chemocauterizing agents, such as trichloroacetic acid or podophyllin, is no longer used in most practices because of their lack of efficacy.

Patient-provided therapies can be used off-label to treat the lesions caused by molluscum contagiosum. Imiquimod 5 % cream has been shown to be an effective and safe therapy when applied once daily, 5 days a week for 4–16 weeks [54] to people with lesions that are resistant to standard therapies. In another study with imiquimod 5 % cream, given only 3 days a week (every other day) for a maximum of 16 weeks, lesions in 78 % of study completers cleared completely [55]. Potassium hydroxide 5–10 % can be applied twice a day to each of the lesions with a swab. Resolution occurs in a mean of 30 days [56]. Other agents that have been reported to have efficacy include cidofovir topically applied, cimetidine orally, iodine solution and salicylic acid plaster, and tape stripping [57].

Partner Notification and Reporting Requirements

Sexual partners should be examined and treated if lesions are present. There are no reporting requirements.

Pregnancy-Related Issues

Molluscum Contagiosum is not known to have any adverse impact on pregnancy.

References

1. Schwartz DA. Lymphogranuloma venereum. In: Connor DH, Chandler FW, Schwartz DA, Mantz HJ, Lack EE, editors. Pathology of infectious diseases. Stamford, CT: Appleton & Lange; 1997. p. 491–7.

2. Blank S, Schillinger JA, Harbatkin D. Lymphogranuloma venereum in the industrialised world. Lancet. 2005;365:1607–8.
3. Sweet RL, Gibbs RS. Sexually transmitted diseases. In: Infectious diseases of the female genital tract. Philadelphia, PA: Lippincott Williams & Wilkins, 2002, pp. 118–175.
4. Bolan RK, Sands M, Schachter J, Miner RC, Drew WL. Lymphogranuloma venereum and acute ulcerative proctitis. Am J Med. 1982;72:703–6.
5. Bauwens JE, Lampe MF, Suchland RJ, Wong K, Stamm WE. Infection with Chlamydia trachomatis lymphogranuloma venereum serovar L1 in homosexual men with proctitis: molecular analysis of an unusual case cluster. Clin Infect Dis. 1995;20:576–81. http://ladhs.org/wps/portal.
6. Centers for Disease Control and Prevention. Sexually transmitted diseases treatment guidelines, 2006. MMWR Recomm Rep 2006; 55(RR-11):15,16,20–22. http://www.cdc.gov/std/treatment/. Accessed Nov. 24, 2006.
7. County of Los Angeles Department of Health Services. Provider alert: lymphogranuloma venereum infections in California. Public's Health 2005;5(3):1–2. http://www.ladhs.org/media/tph/TPHMarch2005.pdf. Accessed Nov. 24, 2006.
8. Schachter J, Smith DE, Dawson CR, et al. Lymphogranuloma venereum. I. Comparison of the Frei test, complement fixation test, and isolation of the agent. J Infect Dis. 1969;120:372–5.
9. Koo D, Wetterhall SF. History and current status of the National Notifiable Diseases Surveillance System. J Public Health Manag Pract. 1996;2:4–10.
10. Ducrey A. Experimentelle Untersuchungen uber den Ansteckungsstof des weichen Schankers und uber die Bubonen. Monatsh Prakt Dermatol. 1889;9:387–405.
11. Bezancon F, Griffin V, LeSourd L. Culture du bacille du chancre mou. C R Seances Soc Biol Fil. 1900;52:1048–51.
12. Lewis DA. Diagnostic tests for chancroid. Sex Transm Infect. 2000;76:137–41.
13. Fleming DT, Wasserheit JN. From epidemiological synergy to public health policy and practice: the contribution of other sexually transmitted diseases to sexual transmission of HIV infection. Sex Transm Infect. 1999;75:3–17.
14. Spinola SM, Bauer ME, Munson Jr RS. Immunopathogenesis of Haemophilus ducreyi infection (chancroid). Infect Immun. 2002;70:1667–76.
15. World Health Organization (WHO). Sexually transmitted infections fact sheet. Geneva, Switzerland: WHO; 2004. www.who.int/reproductive-health/rtis/docs/sti_factsheet_2004.pdf. Accessed April 18, 2005.
16. Nikolaidis G, Rosen T. Chancroid. In: Connor DH, Chandler FW, Schwartz DA, Mantz HJ, Lack EE, editors. Pathology of infectious diseases. Stamford, CT: Appleton & Lange; 1997. p. 469–71.
17. Crowe MA, Hall MA. Chancroid. Updated 2005. www.emedicine.com/derm/topic71.htm. Accessed Nov 24, 2006.
18. Ronald AR, Albritton W. Chancroid and Haemophilus ducreyi. In: Holmes KK, Mardh P-A, Sparling PF, et al., editors. Sexually transmitted diseases. New York, NY: McGraw-Hill; 1999. p. 515–23.
19. Plummer FA, D'Costa LJ, Nsanze H, Dylewski J, Karasira P, Ronald AR. Epidemiology of chancroid and Haemophilus ducreyi in Nairobi, Kenya. Lancet. 1983;2:1293–5.
20. Brunham RC. Epidermiology of sexually transmitted diseases in developing countries. In: Wasserheit J, Aral S, Holmes KK, editors. Research issues in human behavior and STDs in the AIDS era. Washington: American Society of Microbiology; 1991. p. 61–80.
21. Al-Tawfiq JA, Thornton AC, Katz BP, et al. Standardization of the experimental model of Haemophilus ducreyi infection in human subjects. J Infect Dis. 1998;178:1684–7.
22. Lockett AE. Serum-free media for the isolation of Haemophilus ducreyi. Lancet. 1991;338:326.
23. Orle KA, Gates CA, Martin DH, Body BA, Weiss JB. Simultaneous PCR detection of Haemophilus ducreyi, Treponema pallidum, and herpes simplex virus types 1 and 2 from genital ulcers. J Clin Microbiol. 1996;34:49–54.
24. Chapel TA, Brown WJ, Jeffres C, Stewart JA. How reliable is the morphological diagnosis of penile ulcerations? Sex Transm Dis. 1977;4:150–2.

25. Dangor Y, Ballard RC, da L Exposto F, Fehler G, Miller SD, Koornhof HJ. Accuracy of clinical diagnosis of genital ulcer disease. Sex Transm Dis 1990; 17:184–9.
26. Lewis DA. Chancroid: clinical manifestations, diagnosis, and management. Sex Transm Infect. 2003;79:68–71.
27. World Health Organization (WHO). Program for sexually transmitted diseases, global program on AIDS. Recommendations for the management of sexually transmitted diseases. WHO/GPA/TEM/94. Geneva: WHO, 1994. http://www.cdph.ca.gov/pubsforms/Guidelines/Documents/CA-STD-Screening-Recommendations.pdf.
28. Bogaerts J, Vuylsteke B, Martinez Tello W, et al. Simple algorithms for the management of genital ulcers: evaluation in a primary health care centre in Kigali, Rwanda. Bull World Health Organ. 1995;73:761–7.
29. California STD/HIV Prevention Training Center. California STD treatment guidelines for adults and adolescents, 2010. Revised January 2010. http://www.cdph.ca.gov/pubsforms/Guidelines/Documents/CA-STD-Screening-Recommendations.pdf. Accessed Nov. 24, 2006.
30. Majmudar B. Granuloma inguinale. In: Connor DH, Chandler FW, Schwartz DA, Mantz HJ, Lack EE, editors. Pathology of infectious diseases. Appleton & Lange: Stamford, CT; 1997. p. 1565–70.
31. Droegemueller W. Infections of the lower genital tract. In: Stenchever MA, Droegemueller W, Herbst AL, Mishell DR, editors. Comprehensive gynecology. 4th ed. St. Louis, MO: Mosby; 2001. p. 641–706.
32. O'Farrell N. Donovanosis. Sex Transm Infect. 2002;78:452–7.
33. Merianos A, Gilles M, Chuah J. Ceftriaxone in the treatment of chronic donovanosis in central Australia. Genitourin Med. 1994;70:84–9.
34. Richens J. The diagnosis and treatment of donovanosis (granuloma inguinale). Genitourin Med. 1991;67:441–52.
35. Kuberski T. Granuloma inguinale (donovanosis). Sex Transm Dis. 1980;7:29–36.
36. Carter J, Bowden FJ, Sriprakash KS, Bastian I, Kemp DJ. Diagnostic polymerase chain reaction for donovanosis. Clin Infect Dis. 1999;28:1168–9.
37. Carter JS, Kemp DJ. A colorimetric detection system for Calymmatobacterium granulomatis. Sex Transm Infect. 2000;76:134–6.
38. Sehgal VN, Prasad AL. Donovanosis. Current concepts. Int J Dermatol. 1986;25:8–16.
39. Govender D, Naidoo K, Chetty R. Granuloma inguinale (donovanosis): an unusual cause of otitis media and mastoiditis in children. Am J Clin Pathol. 1997;108:510–4.
40. Brown ST, Nalley JF, Kraus SJ. Molluscum contagiosum. Sex Transm Dis. 1981;8:227–34.
41. Taillac PP, Bretz S. Molluscum contagiosum. http://www.emedicine.com/emerg/topic317.htm. Accessed Nov. 24, 2006.
42. Postlethwaite R. Molluscum contagiosum. Arch Environ Health. 1970;21:432–52.
43. Gottlieb SL, Myskowski PL. Molluscum contagiosum. Int J Dermatol. 1994;33:453–61.
44. Tyring SK. Molluscum contagiosum: the importance of early diagnosis and treatment. Am J Obstet Gynecol. 2003;189:S12–6.
45. Billstein SA, Mattaliano Jr VJ. The "nuisance" sexually transmitted diseases: molluscum contagiosum, scabies, and crab lice. Med Clin North Am. 1990;74:1487–505.
46. Bugert JJ, Darai G. Recent advances in molluscum contagiosum virus research. Arch Virol Suppl. 1997;13:35–47.
47. Fenner F. Poxviruses. In: Fields BN, Knipe DM, editors. Virology. 2nd ed. New York, NY: New York Press; 1990.
48. Henao M, Freeman RG. Inflammatory molluscum contagiosum. Clinicopathological study of seven cases. Arch Dermatol. 1964;90:479–82.
49. Cockerell CJ. Poxvirus infections. In: Connor DH, Chandler FW, Schwartz DA, Mantz HJ, Lack EE, editors. Pathology of infectious diseases. Stamford, CT: Appleton & Lange; 1997. p. 273–9.
50. Janniger CK, Schwartz RA. Molluscum contagiosum in children. Cutis. 1993;52:194–6.

51. Hughes PS. Treatment of molluscum contagiosum with the 585-nm pulsed dye laser. Dermatol Surg. 1998;24:229–30.
52. Becker TM, Blout JH, Douglas J, Judson FM. Trends in molluscum contagiosum. Dermatol Ther. 2000;13:285–9.
53. Silverberg NB, Sidbury R, Mancini AJ. Childhood molluscum contagiosum: experience with cantharidin therapy in 300 patients. J Am Acad Dermatol. 2000;43:503–7.
54. Hengge UR, Esser S, Schultewolter T, et al. Self-administered topical 5% imiquimod for the treatment of common warts and molluscum contagiosum. Br J Dermatol. 2000;143:1026–31.
55. Liota E, Smith KJ, Buckley R, Menon P, Skelton H. Imiquimod therapy for molluscum contagiosum. J Cutan Med Surg. 2000;4:76–82.
56. Romiti R, Ribeiro AP, Grinblat BM, Rivitti EA, Romiti N. Treatment of molluscum contagiosum with potassium hydroxide: a clinical approach in 35 children. Pediatr Dermatol. 1999;16:228–31.
57. Hanson D, Diven DG. Molluscum contagiosum. Dermatol Online J. 2003;9:2.

Chapter 11
Ectoparasites: Scabies and Pediculosis Pubis

Jo Ann Woodward

Introduction

Scabies has existed for more than 2,500 years. It was described in ancient texts from the Middle East, China, and India [1]. The word "scabies" is believed to have originated from scabere, the Latin term meaning "to scratch." It was not until 1687 that Bonomo and Cestoni described the casual relationship between the mite and the disease [2]. More than 300 million cases of scabies are diagnosed each year. It is a sexually transmitted infection (STI), but it can be spread by other activities that involve close personal skin contact. The pruritus caused by the infestation is very distressing in itself, but the burrows directly caused by the mite and the excoriations caused by the scratch also make the host susceptible to secondary skin infection and systemic sepsis.

Infestation with lice is referred to as pediculosis. About 4,000 species of lice exist; only about 560 species suck blood and feed only on mammals; three species infest humans. Phthiriasis (pediculosis pubis) is a lice infestation usually located in the pubic region, commonly called "crabs." *Phthirus pubis* is a blood-sucking louse that is a very successful obligate parasite of humans. Infestations are found in all socioeconomic strata.

Fast Facts

- Scabies is highly contagious and is spread by close personal contact, including sexual contact.
- Lesions from scabies are intensely pruritic but may not be visible.

J.A. Woodward, WHNP-BC (✉)
Scottsdale, AZ 85258, USA
e-mail: npjoann@aol.com

N.S. Skolnik et al. (eds.), *Sexually Transmitted Diseases: A Practical Guide for Primary Care*, Current Clinical Practice, DOI 10.1007/978-1-62703-499-9_11,
© Springer Science+Business Media New York 2013

- Diagnosis of scabies is clinical and can be confirmed by microscopic examination of a skin scraping.
- Treatment for scabies must include treatment of the entire body as well as treatment of clothing and bedding.
- Crusted or Norwegian scabies, which can involve infestation with hundreds of thousands or millions of mites, are more common in immunocompromised hosts.
- Scabies complicated by superinfection can be fatal.
- Pediculosis pubis is more contagious than any other STI.
- *P. pubis* (crab louse) is visible with the naked eye.
- Diagnosis is made if the louse and the nits (eggs) are seen on body hair.
- Thirty percent of patients with pediculosis pubis have another STI.
- Children with crab lice in their eyelashes should be evaluated as potential victims of sexual abuse.
- Pediculosis pubis can involve all hairy parts of the body except the scalp, so treatment should not be restricted to the genital area.
- The louse contains host DNA, which may be helpful in identifying rapists.

Scabies

Prevalence/Incidence

Prevalence of scabies worldwide is not known but it has been estimated that more than 300 million people are infested [3]. Historically, epidemics of scabies occur in times of war, famine, and overcrowding [4]. In the United States and Europe, scabies occurs in cycles every 3 decades. Prevalence is 0–6 % [5]. Individuals under age 20 are more commonly infected, but gender and ethnicity are not risk factors. In developing countries, the infestation is chronic and affects up to 30 % of the population [6]. The disease spreads rapidly in institutions such as correctional facilities, health care facilities, and nursing homes, but is not commonly found in schools. The current epidemic has disproportionately affected people infected with human immunodeficiency virus (HIV).

Transmission/Infection

Scabies is a highly contagious condition. Spread of the scabetic mite ("itch mite") requires direct skin-to-skin contact with an infested person. Occasionally, cases are transmitted by contaminated clothing or bedding. Human and canine scabies mites remain infective at room temperature off the host for only 3 days [7]. Fomites, therefore, are possible, but inefficient, vectors. Mites are attracted by heat and odor to seek out hosts. The mites are motionless at room temperature. They cannot fly or jump, but they can crawl as fast as 1 in. per minute on warm skin [4]. Unlike most

STIs, which can spread by brief sexual contact, scabies is more likely to be transmitted by sharing a bed for a night [8].

Etiology

Scabies is caused by an eight-legged blind mite, *Sarcoptes scabiei*. In the female, the front two legs have suckers and the rear two ones are tipped with bristles, but the male has pods on his last pair of legs to hold the female during mating [9]. *S. scabiei* is an obligate parasite, requiring an appropriate host for survival. It subsists on dissolved human tissue but does not feed on blood [4]. The female mite is shield-shaped and measures in 0.3–0.4 mm; the male mite is half as large. The mites mate on the skin surface. The male mite dies. The female mite burrows beneath the epidermis secreting enzymes that dissolve the skin, which she then ingests. It takes the mite 30 min to enter the skin as she burrows head first using her jaws and cutting claws on her forelegs to create the burrow. The female lays 1–3 eggs each day for the rest of her 4–6-week life span. The egg hatches in 2–4 days as six-legged larvae, which cuts through the burrow roof to reach the skin surface. The larvae hides in the hair follicles and skin folds and progresses through two more developmental phases before then it molts into adults. The adult moves to the skin surface to mate. Less than 1 % of the eggs laid complete this life cycle [10].

Canine mites, which cause mange in dogs, may also attach to humans. The infestation occurs in areas of the body that come in contact with the dog (arms and trunk). The canine mite cannot live on humans, so there are no burrows.

Clinical Manifestation

Scabies presents with intensely pruritic papular rash. The pruritus worsens at night. The initial symptom starts 2–6 weeks after initial infestation and often has a gradual onset. Typically, the patient is infested with 10–15 mites (range 3–50). The pruritus results from a delayed type IV hypersensitivity reaction to the mites, their eggs, saliva, and scybala (pockets of feces) [7]. Patients who are re-infested are already sensitized and develop symptoms in only 1–4 days.

On exam, the mite burrows can be found on the patient's hands, interphalangeal finger webs, wrists, peri-umbilical skin, waistline, and axillary folds. The mites prefer the keratinized skin with a few pilosebaceous follies [9]. The sexually transmitted infestations often involve the penis, scrotum, labia, areola, nipples, and buttocks. In adults, the face and scalp are spared, as are the palms and soles. The back is also usually spared except in bedridden individuals. The burrows are short, thin, elevated, serpiginous, gray-colored tracks. The burrows are often destroyed by scratching and may be difficult to see. At the end of the burrow, a small papule may be found. There is often widespread secondary excoriation, pustules, or crusting.

There are different scabies lesions. The most common is erythematous papular or vesicular lesions that are associated with burrows. They may be bullous or urticarial due to an intense immune response [11, 12]. Other forms include nodular, bullous, and keratotic variations. Nodular scabies, which comprises 10 % of cases, presents with dark pruritic nodules that are 5–20 mm in diameter. The nodules are smooth and red, pink, tan, or brown in color. The nodules spontaneously resolve in weeks or months, but may leave post-inflammatory hyperpigmentation. Keratotic, crusting, or "Norwegian" scabies are variants that most commonly afflict immunocompromised hosts. The lesions are generally more widespread and represent infestation with hundreds of thousands to millions of mites. The lesions are large, hyperkeratotic, warty crusts that are filled with burrows, which can last for years. The areas under the fingernails are filled with debris; the palms and soles show deep fissuring of the crusts. Because these hosts are not able to mount an inflammatory reaction, there is less pruritus associated with keratotic scabies. A second type of lesion seen in scabies is a generalized papular eruptions not located in the area of the mite. The papules are formed on the trunk and thighs. They appear erythematous and are thought to be an allergic response to the mite [13].

The classical presentations are not always seen. It takes 4–6 weeks to demonstrate a primary infestation. Early infestations are difficult to detect because the lesions are scarce; the burrows are only 5 mm long and may be difficult to visualize. Wide and sparse lesions may also be seen in patients using systemic or topical lesions. Elderly patients may have intense itching without a visible inflammatory response. Often the excoriation can reduce the number of mites and either obscure or destroy the burrows. In long-standing scabies infections, the skin has a more eczematous appearance. If the secondary infection develops, the lesions look pustular.

Scabies is generally self-limiting in humans. However, untreated scabies can become superinfected, which can lead to cellulitis, abscesses, sepsis, and glomerulonephritis [14]. Because the mites and the mite fecal pellets contain streptococcus and staphylococci, it is possible that the mite also contributes to the infection. Secondary infection of scabies with group A streptococcus pyogenes is a major precursor to acute poststreptococcal glomerulonephritis [15, 16].

Diagnosis

Diagnosis can be made empirically based on the history of intense pruritus, which worsens at night, and the presence of characteristic lesions located in areas typically affected by the infestation. If other family members are affected, the diagnosis is even more secure. The lesions can be better visualized with a hand lens. If there is difficulty identifying the burrow, the best method to find them is by staining. The Burrow Ink Test is performed by flooding an area of skin with fountain pen ink, wiping it clean with alcohol, and identifying the wavy burrows that retain the ink

[17]. Liquid tetracycline can be substituted for the ink and Wood's light and magnifying lens are used to visualize the tetracycline-filled burrows.

Microscopic analysis of the infestation may be prudent, particularly when the lesions have atypical appearances. In order to obtain a specimen, gently scrape the roof off five or six burrows with an oil-covered blunt scalpel blade; the oil will help the material adhere to the blade. The best sites to examine are new, nonexcoriated burrows in the skin webs between the fingers. Place the material on a glass slide. Add a drop of mineral oil or 10 % potassium hydroxide and study the specimen under low power. Visualizing the mite, eggs, or egg shells confirms the diagnosis. Video dermatoscopy is an effective and sensitive diagnostic tool, which allows in vivo visualization of the skin with magnification up to 600 times [4].

Treatment

The Centers for Disease Control and Prevention (CDC) treatment guidelines are outlined in 2010 STD Guidelines—MMWR Recommendations and Reports Dec 17, 2010 [22]. Careful selection of the correct topical agent depends on the patient's age, pregnancy status, and skin condition. Permethrin cream 5 % is a widely used synthetic pyrethroid insecticide whose parent compound was derived from chrysanthemums [18]. It is poorly absorbed through the skin and well-tolerated. It should be applied from the neck down and washed off after 8–14 h. Ivermectin is a macrocyclic lactone antibiotic that is given orally in two doses 1 week apart. Lindane is not recommended as first-line therapy because of toxicity. Lindane is an organochloride insecticide to which the mites have shown some resistance. In addition, it can be absorbed through the skin (especially directly after bathing or through damaged skin) and cause severe neurotoxicity and aplastic anemia. It should be washed off 8 h after application. Bedding and clothing require attention. Because the mites cannot survive more than 3 days without a host, isolating the materials for 72 h will kill all the mites. However, machine washing or drying on a hot cycle will also kill any mites on clothing or bedding immediately. Trimming fingernails helps reduce the potential injury from scratching. The pruritus and inflammation in scabies can be treated with antihistamines or steroids [7]. Additional dosing is needed to treat keratotic (crusting or "Norwegian") scabies because the magnitude of infestations is so impressive. Combined therapies with topical and oral agents or repeated treatment with oral agents has been suggested by experts.

It should be noted that the pruritus might persist for up to 2 weeks after effective eradication of the infestation. However, if symptoms persist beyond 14 days, the diagnosis should be reevaluated. It is also possible that the treatment was applied incorrectly or that reinfestation has occurred [19]. Resistance, particularly to lindane, has been well-documented [20].

Partner Notification and Reporting Requirements

Both sexual and close personal and household contacts within the preceding month should be examined and treated for scabies. Scabies is not a reportable disease.

Special Pregnancy-Related Issues

The CDC recommended treatment in pregnant and breastfeeding women is perme-thrin. Permethrin has been rated (BM) compatible in pregnancy and breastfeeding by other experts [21]. Those same experts rate lindane a category BM drug (limited human data but animal suggest low-risk manufacturer rating), but because of lin-dane's potentially serious neurotoxicity, the CDC states that it should not be used for pregnant or lactating women [22]. The CDC recommends that Ivermectin not be used in lactating women, but the American Academy of Pediatrics classifies Ivermectin as compatible with breastfeeding [23].

Pediculosis Pubis

Prevalence and Incidence

It has been estimated that three million cases of pediculosis pubis are treated each year in the United States [8]. Pediculosis pubis most commonly infests adults and young adults. In the 15–19-year-old age group, women are more likely to be infested than men are. Over age 20, men are more likely to be infested [24].

Transmission and Infectivity

Pubic lice infestation is generally classified as an STI. Transmission occurs most commonly by close physical contact, such as sexual intercourse or sleeping in the same bed. The infection is more contagious than any other STI, with a 95 % chance of contacting the infestation after only one single sexual encounter [25]. However, fomite transmission is also possible by sharing towels or underwear. Condoms do not prevent the transmission of pediculosis pubis.

Etiology

P. pubis (the crab louse) is one of three types of lice that uniquely infest humans and are generally site-specific. The crab louse measures 0.8–1.2 mm in length and width. It is tough-skinned and gray-brown in color (but turns rusty color after feeding). It is a wingless, dorsoventrally flattened louse. The louse has six-paired clawed legs, the last two pairs that are adapted to grasp widely spaced pubic hair. The front pair of legs is shortened. Lice pierce the skin every few hours to obtain a blood meal. The louse inserts its mouth parts into the skin and injects saliva that has vasodilating properties to facilitate access to the blood. Crab lice move 10 cm per day [26]. Within 24 h after mating, the female starts to lay about four eggs per day. The eggs are laid on hair near the root and cemented in a characteristic angle from that strand. The nits incubate for 7 days, after which time a nymph hatches. The nymph proceeds through three moltings in the next 8–9 days and enters into the adult phase. The life span of the female adult crab louse is about 17 days; for the male, it is 22 days [7]. *P. pubis* can live away from the host for about 2 days [4].

Clinical Presentation

The incubation time of pediculosis pubis is 30 days. People generally will present with pruritus, irritation, and/or rash. The pruritus is owing to allergic sensitivity [25]. Patients may also have papular urticaria and excoriation. Occasionally, patients will seek care because they see the louse moving over the skin or along the hair follicle. If the patient suffers large numbers of bites in a short time of period, he or she may have low-grade fevers, malaise, or irritability.

The lice, nits, and excoriation are hallmarks of infestations. For longer-standing infestations, another characteristic finding is maculae ceruleau, which are bluish-gray macules found on the skin of the lower abdomen and thighs from the bites of the *P. pubis*. The color of the macules is assumed to be related to hemosiderin deposits in the deep dermis. Patients may also note some spots of blood or crusting in their underwear.

Pubic lice are not limited to the pubic region. They may be found in other short hairs of the body, such as facial, back, chest, or thigh hairs; eyebrows; eyelashes; and hair at the scalp line. Infestation in the eyelashes is called pediculosis ciliaris. Atypical locations are more common if the pubic region was already locally treated [17].

Diagnosis

The diagnosis of pediculosis pubis can be made if the louse or the nits (lice egg cases) are seen with the naked eye. Identification of the nits may be facilitated with the use of a hand-held magnifying lens. Pluck suspicious-looking hairs and examine in mineral oil under the microscope. It may be possible to differentiate the pubic lice nits from the hair louse nit. The pubic lice nits are attached to the hair shaft at a relatively more acute angle [26]. Nits on the pubic hairs may be confused with white piedra or trichomycosis pubis. Excoriation may result from concurrent infestation with scabies or contact dermatitis.

The diagnosis of pediculosis pubis should prompt testing for other STIs. Thirty percent of individuals with pubic lice have another concurrent STI and, therefore, should undergo screening for HIV, syphilis, gonorrhea, *Chlamydia*, herpes, warts, and trichomoniasis [26]. Children with *P. pubis* in the eyelashes should be evaluated for sexual abuse.

Treatment

The pubic louse is totally encased in a proteinaceous sheath (except for the orifice through which it feeds). As a result, it is more resistant to topical therapies than are other lice. The CDC treatment recommendations are displayed in 2010 STD Guidelines—MMWR Recommendations and Reports Dec 17, 2010 [22]. Each is a rinse or shampoo, which must be applied to the pubic areas and all other affected areas and later rinsed off as directed. Infestation in the eyelashes should not be treated with any of the recommended regimens. Pediculosis of the eyelids should be treated by applying occlusive ophthalmic ointment (such as Vaseline petroleum jelly) twice a day for 10 days. Patients with pediculosis pedis should be evaluated for other STIs.

Bedding and clothing should be decontaminated. Decontamination can be done actively with machine washing and drying using hot cycles or dry cleaning, or passively by removing it from body contact for 72 h, during which time all the pubic lice will die. Fumigation of living areas is not necessary.

If symptoms persist, the patient should be reevaluated after 1 week. Retreatment may be necessary if lice are found or if eggs are observed at the hair–skin junction. Patients who do not respond to a recommended therapy should be retreated with an alternative regimen.

Treatment must include the patient's sex partner(s) within the last month. Sexual and other close contact with partner(s) should be avoided until both partners have been treated and reevaluated after 1 week to rule out persistent disease.

If pubic lice infestation is diagnosed in a sexual assault investigation, there may be enough blood in a single louse to identify a rapist's DNA by polymerase chain reaction. Mechanical removal of as many lice as possible may be important to obtain evidence [26].

Partner Notification and Reporting Requirements

Partners in the last month should be contacted and treated. Partners should also be tested for other STIs. There is no uniform requirement to report *P. pubis* to the local public health department.

Pregnancy-Related Issues

Pregnant and lactating women should be treated with either permethrin or pyrethrin with piperonyl butoxide. The CDC says that lindane is contraindicated for use by pregnant or breastfeeding women.

Case Study

Pat is a 23-year-old graduate student who presents with intense pruritus in her pelvic area. She had initially thought that she had a yeast infection; she treated herself with an over-the-counter antifungal cream, but the itching got worse. Her last menstrual period started 5 weeks ago. She received her first injection of depomedroxyprogesterone acetate 3 days later. She is in a fairly stable relationship with her boyfriend except one episode just before her last period, when she and her boyfriend had a fight. She slept with a former partner and thinks they used condoms. On exam, she has an impressive infestation of *P. pubis*.

Questions

1. Would you require her to have a pregnancy test before administering drug therapy?
2. Does she need any other tests?
3. Who should be tested and treated? For which infection(s)?
4. What other measures does she need to take?
5. What if she is still symptomatic in a week?

Answers

1. It is highly unlikely that she is pregnant, given that she had a timely injection of depo-medroxyprogesterone acetate. Because the first-line treatment is permethrin, there is no need to do pregnancy testing.
2. She needs testing for at least *Chlamydia* and a microscopic assessment to rule out vaginal infections. HIV testing in a month might also be prudent. Other STI tests may also be indicated once more history about the infecting partner is obtained.

3. All of her sexual contacts in the last month should be examined and treated for *P. pubis* and tested for other STIs.
4. Her bedding and clothing must be decontaminated. She must not have intimate contact until 1 week after she and her partner have both been treated.
5. If she is symptomatic 1 week after therapy, consider reexposure. If she has a resistant infection, she may need to be treated with lindane. A pregnancy test would be needed before this therapy. All of her sexual contacts who were treated would also have to be reevaluated for their response to therapy.

References

1. Alexander JO'D. Scabies. In: Arthropods and human skin. Berlin: Springer; 1984. p. 227–92.
2. Parish LC. History of scabies. In: Orkin M, Maibach HI, Parish LC, Schwartzman RM, editors. Scabies and pediculosis. Philadelphia, PA: Lippincott; 1977. p. 1–6.
3. Taplin D, Meinking TL, Chen JA, Sanchez R. Comparison of crotamiton 10 % cream (Eurax) and permethrin 5 % cream (Elimite) for the treatment of scabies in children. Pediatr Dermatol. 1990;7:67–73.
4. Steen CJ, Carbonaro PA, Schwartz RA. Arthropods in dermatology. J Am Acad Dermatol. 2004;50:819–42; quiz 842–4.
5. Epstein E, Orkin M. Scabies: clinical aspects. In: Orkin M, Maibach HI, editors. Cutaneous infestations and insect bites. New York, NY: Marcel Decker; 1985. p. 19–24.
6. Burkhart CG. Scabies: an epidemiologic reassessment. Ann Intern Med. 1983;98:498–503.
7. Huynh TH, Norman RA. Scabies and pediculosis. Dermatol Clin. 2004;22:7–11.
8. Sweet RL, Gibbs RS. Sexually transmitted diseases. In: Sweet RL, Gibbs RS, editors. Infectious diseases of the female genital tract. 4th ed. Philadelphia, PA: Lippincott Williams & Wilkins; 2001. p. 118–75.
9. Conner DH. Scabies. In: Conner DH, Chandler FW, Schwartz DA, Manz HJ, Lack EE, editors. Pathology of infectious diseases. Stamford, CT: Appleton and Lange; 1997. p. 1695–8.
10. Mellanby K. Scabies in 1976. R Soc Health J. 1977;97:32–36, 40.
11. Witkowski JA, Parish LC. Scabies. Subungual areas harbor mites. JAMA. 1984;252:1318–9.
12. Chapel TA, Krugel L, Chapel J, Segal A. Scabies presenting as urticaria. JAMA. 1981;246:1440–1.
13. Mellanby K. Scabies. 2nd ed. Hampton: EW Classey; 1972.
14. Burgess I. Sarcoptes scabiei and scabies. Adv Parasitol. 1994;33:235–92.
15. Svartman M, Finklea JF, Earle DP, Potter EV, Poon-King T. Epidemic scabies and acute glomerulonephritis in Trinidad. Lancet. 1972;1:249–51.
16. Hersch C. Acute glomerulonephritis due to skin disease, with special reference to scabies. S Afr Med J. 1967;41:29–34.
17. Woodley D, Saurat JH. The Burrow Ink Test and the scabies mite. J Am Acad Dermatol. 1981;4:715–22.
18. McCarthy JS, Kemp DJ, Walton SF, Currie BJ. Scabies: more than just an irritation. Postgrad Med J. 2004;80:382–7.
19. Karthikeyan K. Treatment of scabies: newer perspectives. Postgrad Med J. 2005;81:7–11.
20. Boix V, Sanchez-Paya J, Portilla J, Merino E. Nosocomial outbreak of scabies clinically resistant to lindane. Infect Control Hosp Epidemiol. 1997;18:677.
21. Briggs GG, Freeman RK, Yaffe SJ, editors. Drugs in pregnancy and lactation: a reference guide to fetal and neonatal risk. 7th ed. Baltimore, MD: Williams & Wilkins; 2005.

22. Centers for Disease Control and Prevention. 2010 STD Guidelines. MMWR recommendations and reports Dec 17, 2010; Vol 59:RR. http://www.cdc.gov/std/treatment/. Accessed Feb 20, 2013.
23. American Academy of Pediatrics Committee on Drugs. Transfer of drugs and other chemicals into human milk. Pediatrics. 2001;108:776–89.
24. Fisher I, Morton RS. Phthirus pubis infestation. Br J Vener Dis. 1970;46:326–9.
25. Felman YM, Nikitas JA. Pediculosis pubis. Cutis 1980; 25:482, 487–489, 559.
26. Ko CJ, Elston DM. Pediculosis. J Am Acad Dermatol. 2004;50:1–12.

Chapter 12
Public Health and Prevention

Elissa Meites and Kimberly A. Workowski

Introduction

Sexually transmitted diseases (STDs) are a challenging public health problem with tremendous health and economic impacts. In the United States alone, there are approximately 20 million new sexually transmitted infections per year [1], and the estimated annual direct medical cost is $16 billion [2]. Of all the notifiable infectious diseases in the United States, the one most commonly reported is chlamydia [3]. Most sexually active persons will have at least one sexually transmitted infection during their lifetime, though many will never know it [1, 4–6].

STD epidemics encompass behavioral, biomedical, and sociopolitical realities. Although STDs can affect people of all races and ethnicities, ages, and geographic areas, marginalized populations may be particularly vulnerable to the consequences of disease. STD prevention is all the more challenging due to the effects of cultural taboos, stigma, and discrimination. STD outbreaks can reveal vulnerabilities in a community's access to appropriate medical care, quality education and health information, healthy economic and social policies, and other structural failures [7].

E. Meites, MD, MPH, FAAFP (✉)
Division of STD Prevention, Centers for Disease Control and Prevention, Atlanta, GA, USA
e-mail: emeites@cdc.gov

K.A. Workowski, MD, FIDSA, FACP
Division of STD Prevention, Centers for Disease Control and Prevention, Atlanta, GA, USA

Department of Medicine, Infectious Diseases, Emory University, Atlanta, GA, USA

N.S. Skolnik et al. (eds.), *Sexually Transmitted Diseases: A Practical Guide for Primary Care*, Current Clinical Practice, DOI 10.1007/978-1-62703-499-9_12, © Springer Science+Business Media New York 2013

Table 12.1 Epidemiology of selected sexually transmitted infections compared with their status as nationally notifiable infectious conditions in the United States

Infection	Nationally notifiable [47]	Epidemiology [1]
Human papillomavirus (HPV)	No	Prevalence: 24 million persons
Herpes simplex virus (HSV) type 2	No	Prevalence: 79 million persons
Trichomoniasis	No	Prevalence: 3.7 million persons
Chlamydia	Yes	Annual incidence: 2.9 million cases
Gonorrhea	Yes	Annual incidence: 820,000 cases
Syphilis	Yes	Annual incidence: 55,000 cases
Chancroid	Yes	Annual incidence: 24 cases [8]

Public Health Information

Public health organizations in the United States include health departments in every state, as well as the Centers for Disease Control and Prevention (CDC) at the national level. Public health activities of particular value to clinicians include surveillance for trends in who is acquiring infections and diseases, or trends in antimicrobial resistance. Local and state health departments may collect case reports of certain diseases, conduct partner notification and contact tracing during investigations of communicable diseases, and provide clinical consultation and education. Nationally, there are federally funded STD control programs for chlamydia, gonorrhea, and syphilis. In addition to providing leadership and financial support, key functions of public health organizations at the state and national levels are to guide research and policy development, and to assess, provide, and interpret timely scientific information regarding STDs.

Information about the epidemiology (prevalence and incidence) of STDs in the US population is derived from several different sources. These include (A) surveillance of reportable diseases; (B) nationally representative surveys; and (C) studies in special populations. Although the most commonly reported diseases are STDs, the most common sexually transmitted infections are not nationally notifiable (Table 12.1).

First, surveillance occurs for certain conditions which are considered to be of public health importance. While state policies vary regarding which conditions are reportable, the nationally notifiable STDs are chancroid, chlamydia, gonorrhea, and syphilis (Table 12.1). In addition, viral hepatitis and HIV are also notifiable conditions but are not always sexually transmitted. Case reports may be generated from a clinician who makes the diagnosis, a laboratory where a clinical test is positive, or a local health department following the case; reports are transmitted to the state health department. Each state health department then provides CDC with the overall numbers of cases to create the national surveillance estimates, which are compiled and published annually [3, 8].

Second, studies conducted on a nationally representative sample can provide helpful estimates of the prevalence of STDs that are common but not reportable. One example is the National Health and Nutrition Examination Survey (NHANES), a population-based study conducted on a representative sample of the civilian, noninstitutionalized population of the United States. Estimates of the national prevalence of common infections such as human papillomavirus (HPV), genital herpes, and trichomoniasis can be extrapolated from the prevalence detected in NHANES participants [9].

Third, special studies are useful to measure STDs in specific at-risk or minority populations, such as adolescents, pregnant women, men who have sex with men, and others. These types of studies are also useful to learn about less common conditions such as neonatal herpes, pelvic inflammatory disease (PID), or lymphogranuloma venereum. All research studies involving human subjects receive additional oversight from institutional review boards (IRBs) to ensure that the research conducted is ethical and its methods are sound.

Public Health and Clinicians

To improve population health, however, public health efforts rely on the foundation of the clinical encounter. Clinicians observe and assess symptoms and signs, request laboratory tests, make a diagnosis, and offer interactive counseling for individual patients. Primary care providers in particular play a unique and important role in routine sexual history-taking, risk assessment, and risk reduction counseling.

To help guide clinicians, CDC produces national STD treatment guidelines, which offer recommendations on the prevention, diagnosis, and treatment of STDs and sexually transmitted infections [10]. Clinically, the prevention and control of STDs are based on five major strategies:

- Education and counseling of persons at risk on ways to avoid STDs through changes in sexual behaviors and use of recommended prevention strategies (e.g., condoms).
- Screening and identification of asymptomatically infected persons and of symptomatic persons unlikely to seek diagnostic and treatment services.
- Effective diagnosis, treatment, and counseling of infected persons.
- Evaluation, treatment, and counseling of sex partners of persons who are infected with an STD.
- Pre-exposure vaccination of persons at risk for vaccine-preventable STDs (e.g., hepatitis A, hepatitis B, HPV).

Public Health Problems in STD Control and Prevention

The following examples of major public health problems will highlight the crucial role of clinicians and discuss how the above strategies can help prevention and control of STDs. Major problems include antimicrobial-resistant gonorrhea, STD-related cancers, STD-related HIV acquisition and transmission, STD-related infertility, and STD-related adverse outcomes of pregnancy.

Antimicrobial-Resistant Neisseria gonorrhoeae

There are estimated to be over 820,000 new cases of gonorrhea in the United States each year [1]. The epidemiology of gonorrhea varies greatly among communities, and disproportionately affects certain populations, including adolescents and young adults, blacks, and men who have sex with men [8]. Untreated gonorrheal infections can lead to PID and infertility. Most of the time, gonorrhea can be treated successfully using a third-generation cephalosporin antimicrobial. However, gonorrhea treatment has been complicated by the ability of *N. gonorrhoeae* to develop resistance to many antimicrobials over the past several decades. From 2006 through 2010, the minimum concentrations of cefixime needed to inhibit the growth of gonorrhea strains in the United States and many other countries increased, suggesting that the effectiveness of this medication may be waning [11]. These patterns may indicate the impending development of clinically significant gonococcal resistance to cephalosporins [11].

Priorities for clinicians include treating all cases of gonorrhea with the most effective available antimicrobial regimen, as well as offering male latex condoms, risk-reduction counseling and testing for other STDs. Due to the possibility of reinfection, repeat gonorrhea testing 3 months following appropriate treatment at the anatomic site of infection is recommended [10]. In addition, providers should ensure that all sex partners from the preceding 60 days are promptly evaluated and treated. Primary screening should be targeted and offered to persons who are considered to be at increased risk, taking into consideration the local prevalence of gonorrhea [12, 13]. Due to the widespread use of nucleic acid amplification tests for gonorrhea diagnosis, laboratory capacity to isolate *N. gonorrhoeae* by culture has been declining; healthcare systems should support continued access to culture or develop partnerships with laboratories that can perform culture. Local, state, and national public health organizations can provide helpful consultation.

STD-Related Cancers

Cervical cancers are caused by certain types of HPV, particularly HPV types 16 and 18. In addition, many anal cancers, oropharyngeal cancers, vulvar, and penile cancers are caused by HPV, although the natural history and epidemiology of these cancers have been less fully described [14].

HPV is a common infection in both men and women, and first infection can occur soon after sexual debut [15, 16]. Virtually all sexually active persons will be infected with at least one type of HPV at some point during their lives [4, 5]. An estimated 79 million persons in the United States are currently infected with at least one type of HPV [1]; among 14–59-year-old women, the prevalence of any type of HPV is 42.5 % [17]. Most HPV infections resolve spontaneously without any treatment—about 70 % clear within 1 year, and 90 % within 2 years—however, those that persist can develop into intraepithelial lesions and cancers [18, 19]. The most common kind of HPV-associated cancer is cervical cancer, which affects an estimated 12,000 women each year in the United States; globally, the vast majority of cervical cancer deaths occur in women in developing countries [14, 20]. Men who have sex with men appear to be at particularly high risk for HPV-associated diseases; their incidence of anal cancer is estimated to be 37 times higher than that among men who have sex with only women [21, 22].

Since 2006, HPV vaccine has been routinely recommended in the United States for females at a target age of 11 or 12 years; since 2011, vaccine has been recommended for males at this age as well [23, 24]. Before a vaccine can be used in the United States, it must be licensed by the US Food and Drug Administration (FDA), which requires safety and efficacy data for the vaccine. Next, national vaccine policy is made by the Advisory Committee on Immunization Practices (ACIP), a panel of independent experts organized by the CDC with formal meetings three times a year. ACIP recommendations are based on the best available scientific evidence on the use of the vaccine in populations, such as vaccine efficacy and safety, epidemiology, and burden of disease in the United States, cost and cost-effectiveness, vaccine acceptability, and implementation plans. HPV vaccine is covered by most insurance plans as well as the Vaccines for Children Program in the United States [25]. Vaccination is one of the most effective methods for preventing HPV infection; clinicians should make strong recommendations and vaccinate adolescents on time.

STD-Related HIV Acquisition and Transmission

Not only is the diagnosis of a new sexually transmitted infection an objective marker of unprotected sexual activity, but in addition, certain STDs can increase plasma HIV viral load and genital HIV shedding, which may also increase the risk of sexual and perinatal HIV transmission [10, 26, 27].

Identification of sexual risk behaviors, risk reduction counseling, appropriate diagnosis, and treatment are important in the prevention and management of specific STDs that can increase HIV acquisition and transmission. In particular, STDs that cause ulceration or inflammation (e.g., syphilis, herpes, trichomoniasis, and chancroid) can increase the transmissibility of HIV [28–30]. In the United States, the most common etiologies of genital, anal, or perianal ulceration are genital herpes or syphilis. These infections can be easily confused on physical exam, and laboratory testing is warranted to confirm a specific diagnosis, in order to ensure the correct course of treatment [10].

Genital herpes is a common cause of genital ulceration; in addition, many persons may have mild or unrecognized infection yet shed the virus intermittently. An estimated 24 million people in the United States are infected with herpes simplex virus (HSV) type 2 [1]; more than 80 % of these infections are undiagnosed [31]. A particularly high burden of disease has been observed among non-Hispanic blacks, with a seroprevalence of 39.2 % [31]. The majority of genital herpes infections are transmitted by persons who are unaware of their infection or are asymptomatic when transmission occurs.

Syphilis in the United States tends to cluster geographically and within sexual networks. There are an estimated 55,000 new cases of syphilis annually in the United States [1]; rates among men were more than 7 times higher than among women, and two-thirds of primary and secondary syphilis in men occurred among men who have sex with men [8]. The resurgence of syphilis in patients with HIV infection underscores the importance of primary prevention of syphilis in this population, which should include client-centered risk reduction messages and discussions of specific actions that can reduce the risk of acquiring syphilis and of acquiring or transmitting HIV infection.

Trichomoniasis is quite common, affecting an estimated 3.7 million people in the United States [1], including 3.1 % of women aged 14–49 years [32]. *Trichomonas vaginalis* infection can cause local inflammation that has been associated with an increased risk of HIV acquisition and transmission [32].

Chancroid, an ulcerative STD caused by the bacteria *Haemophilus ducreyi*, has been associated with HIV acquisition [29]. In the United States, prevalence is low: in 2010, only 24 cases of chancroid were reported from nine different states [8].

Because of the likelihood of co-infection, patients who are diagnosed with one STD (or HIV) should also be offered screening for other STDs including HIV, and their sexual partners should be tested and treated as well [10]. In the United States, men who have sex with men may be at particularly high risk of co-infection with both HIV and other STDs. Prompt recognition and appropriate treatment of STDs are important strategies for reducing HIV risk [10].

Studies conducted internationally in high-prevalence areas have shown that male circumcision can also reduce the risk of HIV acquisition in heterosexual men [33]. In addition, recent data has shown effectiveness of antiretroviral therapy for either pre- or postexposure prophylaxis (PrEP and PEP) in reducing acquisition and transmission of HIV [34, 35]. In a double-blind randomized controlled trial, pericoital use of 1 % tenofovir gel reduced HIV-1 acquisition by 39 %, and HSV-2 acquisition by 51 % [36]. Although topical microbicides have been a subject of some interest, trials of agents with nonspecific antimicrobial activity have not proved particularly useful for STD prevention to date [37]. The spermicide nonoxynol-9 (or "N-9") can injure anal and vaginal mucosal tissue and may even enhance HIV transmission [38]. Clinicians can counsel patients on primary prevention methods, including using condoms consistently and correctly, minimizing the number of sexual partners, and avoiding concurrent sexual partnerships [10].

STD-Related Infertility

Gonorrheal and chlamydial infections, even when asymptomatic, can lead to PID and complications including infertility.

Chlamydia is the most commonly reported STD in the United States. Chlamydial infections are usually asymptomatic in women, but can cause significant reproductive health sequelae including acute PID, an important infectious cause of infertility, ectopic pregnancy, and chronic pelvic pain. There are an estimated 2.9 million new cases of chlamydia annually in the United States [1]. Particularly high rates of chlamydia are seen among adolescent girls and women, blacks, and persons in high-risk settings such as juvenile detention facilities, jails, or prisons, as well as STD and family planning clinics [8].

When chlamydial or gonorrheal infections ascend into a woman's upper genital tract, they can induce a host immune response that causes inflammation and tissue damage, which can lead to PID and/or scarring of the fallopian tubes. Long-term consequences can include infertility, ectopic pregnancy, or chronic pelvic pain. An estimated 10 % of women with untreated chlamydia may develop PID, and a proportion of these may go on to develop infertility [39].

Public health programs aim to prevent these reproductive problems before they can occur. Most public health efforts focus on at-risk women, although treating affected male partners is also clinically important. Overlapping public health paradigms focus on (a) preventing initial infections; (b) providing primary screening and treatment for existing infections; and (c) conducting secondary screening for repeat infections [28]. Clinicians play an important role in counseling patients about prevention methods such as using latex condoms consistently and correctly throughout every sexual encounter, and minimizing numbers of sexual partners. In addition, prompt screening and appropriate treatment for chlamydia reduces the risk of PID.

STD-Related Adverse Outcomes of Pregnancy

Many sexually transmitted infections can cause adverse outcomes of pregnancy, including spontaneous abortion, stillbirth, premature delivery, and congenital infections.

Syphilis remains an important cause of infant mortality and morbidity during pregnancy despite availability of serologic screening tests and recommendations for routine prenatal screening and counseling. Thus, each case of congenital syphilis can be seen as a sentinel event, signaling missed opportunities within a health care system. In the United States, congenital syphilis is uncommon, with a total of 377 cases reported from 28 states, the District of Columbia, and one outlying area in 2010 [8].

Genital herpes can also be associated with poor fetal outcomes, especially after primary maternal genital infection acquired in late pregnancy [40]. Neonatal herpes infection is a rare but serious condition caused by HSV; incidence estimates in the United States range from 5.6 to 28.2 per 100,000 births [41, 42]. Guidelines from the American College of Obstetricians and Gynecologists (ACOG) recommend cesarean delivery for women with active genital lesions in order to prevent transmission of HSV to neonates [43]. Although primary prevention is important for women with herpes lesions at the time of delivery, most mothers of infected neonates had asymptomatic HSV infections [44]. Thus, neonatal herpes mitigation also relies on postnatal testing in infants with a compatible clinical presentation, as well as provision of acyclovir antiviral therapy promptly and for an appropriate course of treatment [45, 46].

Other STDs that can result in adverse pregnancy outcomes include gonorrhea, chlamydia, bacterial vaginosis, and trichomoniasis, although data regarding the effects of these infections on pregnancy are more limited. Health care providers can educate and screen pregnant women for gonorrhea and chlamydia per existing guidelines, and also offer treatment and partner services when appropriate [10].

Conclusion

Clinicians can play an important role in the promotion of sexual health and the prevention and control of STDs through the effective use of five major strategies: education and counseling; screening; diagnosis and treatment; partner treatment; and vaccination. Support for clinicians is available from public health organizations at the local, state, and national levels. Communities across the United States rely on multidisciplinary collaboration between clinicians and public health agencies for the prevention and control of major STD-related public health problems.

References

1. Satterwhite CL, Torrone E, Meites E, Dunne EF, Mahajan R, Ocfemia MCB, Su J, Xu F, Weinstock H. Sexually Transmitted Infections among U.S. Women and Men: Prevalence and Incidence Estimates, 2008. Sexually Transmitted Diseases. 2013; 40(3): 187–193. [Research Support, U.S. Gov't].
2. Owusu-Edusei K, Chesson HW, Gift TL, Tao G, Mahajan R, Ocfemia MC, Kent CK. The estimated direct medical cost of selected sexually transmitted infections in the United States, 2008. Sexually Transmitted Diseases. 2013; 40(3):197-201. [Research Support, U.S. Gov't].
3. Centers for Disease Control and Prevention. Summary of notifiable diseases—United States, 2010. MMWR Morb Mortal Wkly Rep. 2012;59(53):1–111.
4. Koutsky L. Epidemiology of genital human papillomavirus infection. Am J Med. 1997;102(5A):3–8 [Review].
5. Myers ER, McCrory DC, Nanda K, Bastian L, Matchar DB. Mathematical model for the natural history of human papillomavirus infection and cervical carcinogenesis. Am J Epidemiol. 2000;151(12):1158–71 [Research Support, U.S. Gov't, P.H.S.].
6. Forhan SE, Gottlieb SL, Sternberg MR, Xu F, Datta SD, McQuillan GM, et al. Prevalence of sexually transmitted infections among female adolescents aged 14 to 19 in the United States. Pediatrics. 2009;124(6):1505–12 [Research Support, U.S. Gov't].
7. Institute of Medicine (U.S.). Committee on Prevention and Control of Sexually Transmitted Diseases, Eng TR, Butler WT. The hidden epidemic: confronting sexually transmitted diseases. Washington DC: National Academy Press; 1997.

8. Centers for Disease Control and Prevention. Sexually transmitted disease surveillance 2010. Atlanta: U.S. Department of Health and Human Services; 2011. http://www.cdc.gov/std/stats/

9. Ezzati TM, Massey JT, Waksberg J, Chu A, Maurer KR. Sample design: Third National Health and Nutrition Examination Survey. Vital Health Stat 2. 1992;113:1–35.

10. Workowski KA, Berman S. Sexually transmitted diseases treatment guidelines, 2010. MMWR Recomm Rep. 2010;59:1–110. http://www.cdc.gov/std/treatment/2010

11. Bolan GA, Sparling PF, Wasserheit JN. The emerging threat of untreatable gonococcal infection. N Engl J Med. 2012;366(6):485–7 [Review].

12. Workowski KA, Berman SM, Douglas Jr JM. Emerging antimicrobial resistance in Neisseria gonorrhoeae: urgent need to strengthen prevention strategies. Ann Intern Med. 2008;148(8):606–13 [Review].

13. Meyers D, Wolff T, Gregory K, Marion L, Moyer V, Nelson H, et al. USPSTF recommendations for STI screening. Am Fam Physician. 2008;77(6):819–24 [Review].

14. Gillison ML, Chaturvedi AK, Lowy DR. HPV prophylactic vaccines and the potential prevention of noncervical cancers in both men and women. Cancer. 2008;113(10 Suppl):3036–46 [Review].

15. Winer RL, Lee SK, Hughes JP, Adam DE, Kiviat NB, Koutsky LA. Genital human papillomavirus infection: incidence and risk factors in a cohort of female university students. Am J Epidemiol. 2003;157(3):218–26 [Research Support, U.S. Gov't].

16. Partridge JM, Hughes JP, Feng Q, Winer RL, Weaver BA, Xi LF, et al. Genital human papillomavirus infection in men: incidence and risk factors in a cohort of university students. J Infect Dis. 2007;196(8):1128–36 [Research Support, N.I.H., Extramural].

17. Hariri S, Unger ER, Sternberg M, Dunne EF, Swan D, Patel S, et al. Prevalence of genital human papillomavirus among females in the United States, the National Health And Nutrition Examination Survey, 2003-2006. J Infect Dis. 2011;204(4):566–73 [Research Support, U.S. Gov't].

18. Molano M, Van den Brule A, Plummer M, Weiderpass E, Posso H, Arslan A, et al. Determinants of clearance of human papillomavirus infections in Colombian women with normal cytology: a population-based, 5-year follow-up study. Am J Epidemiol. 2003;158(5):486–94 [Research Support, Non-U.S. Gov't].

19. Moscicki AB, Shiboski S, Broering J, Powell K, Clayton L, Jay N, et al. The natural history of human papillomavirus infection as measured by repeated DNA testing in adolescent and young women. J Pediatr. 1998;132(2):277–84 [Research Support, Non-U.S. Gov't; Research Support, U.S. Gov't].

20. Paavonen J. Human papillomavirus infection and the development of cervical cancer and related genital neoplasias. Int J Infect Dis. 2007;11 Suppl 2:S3–9 [Review].

21. Joseph DA, Miller JW, Wu X, Chen VW, Morris CR, Goodman MT, et al. Understanding the burden of human papillomavirus-associated anal cancers in the US. Cancer. 2008;113(10 Suppl):2892–900 [Research Support, U.S. Gov't].

22. Seaberg EC, Wiley D, Martinez-Maza O, Chmiel JS, Kingsley L, Tang Y, et al. Cancer incidence in the multicenter AIDS Cohort Study before and during the HAART era: 1984 to 2007. Cancer. 2010;116(23):5507–16 [Comparative Study Research Support, N.I.H., Extramural].

23. Centers for Disease Control and Prevention. Recommendations on the Use of quadrivalent human papillomavirus vaccine in males—Advisory Committee On Immunization Practices (ACIP), 2011. MMWR Morb Mortal Wkly Rep. 2011;60:1705–8.

24. Centers for Disease Control and Prevention. FDA licensure of bivalent human papillomavirus vaccine (HPV2, Cervarix) for use in females and updated HPV vaccination recommendations from the Advisory Committee on Immunization Practices (ACIP). MMWR Morb Mortal Wkly Rep. 2010;59(20):626–9.

25. Centers for Disease Control and Prevention. Progress toward implementation of human papillomavirus vaccination—the Americas, 2006–2010. MMWR Morb Mortal Wkly Rep. 2011;60(40):1382–4.

26. Cohen MS. Classical sexually transmitted diseases drive the spread of HIV-1: back to the future. J Infect Dis. 2012;206(1):1–2 [Review].

27. Hayes R, Watson-Jones D, Celum C, van de Wijgert J, Wasserheit J. Treatment of sexually transmitted infections for HIV prevention: end of the road or new beginning? AIDS. 2010;24 Suppl 4:S15–26 [Research Support, N.I.H., Extramural Research Support, Non-U.S. Gov't].

28. Workowski KA, Levine WC, Wasserheit JN, Centers for Disease Control and Prevention, Atlanta, Georgia. U.S. Centers for Disease Control and Prevention guidelines for the treatment of sexually transmitted diseases: an opportunity to unify clinical and public health practice. Ann Intern Med. 2002;137(4):255–62 [Review].

29. Fleming DT, Wasserheit JN. From epidemiological synergy to public health policy and practice: the contribution of other sexually transmitted diseases. Sex Transm Infect. 1999;75:3–17 [Review].

30. Rottingen JA, Cameron DW, Garnett GP. A systematic review of the epidemiologic interactions between classic sexually transmitted diseases and HIV: how much really is known? Sex Transm Dis. 2001;28:579–97 [Review].

31. Centers for Disease Control and Prevention. Seroprevalence of herpes simplex virus type 2 among persons aged 14–49 years—United States, 2005–2008. MMWR Morb Mortal Wkly Rep. 2010;59(15):456–9.

32. Sutton M, Sternberg M, Koumans EH, McQuillan G, Berman S, Markowitz L. The prevalence of Trichomonas vaginalis infection among reproductive-age women in the United States, 2001-2004. Clin Infect Dis. 2007;45(10):1319–26 [Research Support, U.S. Gov't].

33. Gray RH, Kigozi G, Serwadda D, Makumbi F, Watya S, Nalugoda F, et al. Male circumcision for HIV prevention in men in Rakai, Uganda: a randomised trial. Lancet. 2007;369(9562):657–66 [Randomized Controlled Trial].

34. Smith DK, Grohskopf LA, Black RJ, Auerbach JD, Veronese F, Struble KA, et al. Antiretroviral postexposure prophylaxis after sexual, injection-drug use, or other nonoccupational exposure to HIV in the United States: recommendations from the U.S. Department of Health and Human Services. MMWR Recomm Rep. 2005;54(RR-2):1–20 [Practice Guideline].

35. Centers for Disease Control and Prevention. Interim guidance: preexposure prophylaxis for the prevention of HIV infection in men who have sex with men. MMWR Morb Mortal Wkly Rep. 2011;60(3):65–8.

36. Abdool Karim Q, Abdool Karim SS, Frohlich JA, Grobler AC, Baxter C, Mansoor LE, et al. Effectiveness and safety of tenofovir gel, an antiretroviral microbicide, for the prevention of HIV infection in women. Science. 2010;329(5996):1168–74 [Randomized Controlled Trial; Research Support, N.I.H.; Research Support, Non-U.S. Gov't].

37. Marrazzo JM, Cates W. Interventions to prevent sexually transmitted infections, including HIV infection. Clin Infect Dis. 2011;53 Suppl 3:S64–78 [Review].

38. Phillips DM, Sudol KM, Taylor CL, Guichard L, Elsen R, Maguire RA. Lubricants containing N-9 may enhance rectal transmission of HIV and other STIs. Contraception. 2004;70(2):107–10 [Research Support, U.S. Gov't].

39. Oakeshott P, Kerry S, Aghaizu A, Atherton H, Hay S, Taylor-Robinson D, et al. Randomised controlled trial of screening for Chlamydia trachomatis to prevent pelvic inflammatory disease: the POPI (prevention of pelvic infection) trial. BMJ. 2010;340:c1642 [Multicenter Study; Randomized Controlled Trial; Research Support, Non-U.S. Gov't].

40. Brown ZA, Selke S, Zeh J, Kopelman J, Maslow A, Ashley RL, et al. The acquisition of herpes simplex virus during pregnancy. N Engl J Med. 1997;337(8):509–15.

41. Handel S, Klingler EJ, Washburn K, Blank S, Schillinger JA. Population-based surveillance for neonatal herpes in New York City, April 2006-September 2010. Sex Transm Dis. 2011;38(8):705–11.

42. Flagg EW, Weinstock H. Incidence of neonatal herpes simplex virus infections in the United States, 2006. Pediatrics. 2006;127(1):e1–8 [Research Support, U.S. Gov't].

43. ACOG Committee on Practice Bulletins. ACOG Practice Bulletin. Clinical management guidelines for obstetrician-gynecologists. No. 82 June 2007. Management of herpes in pregnancy. Obstet Gynecol. 2007;109(6):1489–98.

44. Corey L, Wald A. Maternal and neonatal herpes simplex virus infections. N Engl J Med. 2009;361(14):1376–85.
45. Kimberlin DW, Whitley RJ, Wan W, Powell DA, Storch G, Ahmed A, et al. Oral acyclovir suppression and neurodevelopment after neonatal herpes. N Engl J Med. 2011;365(14):1284–92.
46. Shah SS, Aronson PL, Mohamad Z, Lorch SA. Delayed acyclovir therapy and death among neonates with herpes simplex virus infection. Pediatrics. 2011;128(6):1153–60.
47. 2012 Case definitions: nationally notifiable conditions infectious and non-infectious case. Atlanta, GA: Centers for Disease Control and Prevention; 2012 [cited July 11, 2012]. http://www.cdc.gov/osels/ph_surveillance/nndss/phs/infdis2011.htm

Chapter 13
Evaluation and Treatment of STD Exposure and Sexual Assault

Christine M. Stroka and Mathew M. Clark

Introduction

Primary care providers may be asked to evaluate and treat patients who have had unprotected exposure to possible sexually transmitted diseases (STDs). This might occur in a variety of scenarios, ranging from consensual but unprotected sex with a known partner to sexual assault, in which the assailant is unknown.

Because of the unique legal, medical, and psychological issues which arise in the setting of sexual assault, this topic will be addressed in some detail. Many of the principles that apply when a patient has been sexually assaulted are also relevant in addressing other instances of unprotected sex, including preventing pregnancy and empiric treatment for possible STDs. The bulk of information in this chapter is drawn from the Centers for Disease Control and Prevention Sexually Transmitted Diseases Treatment Guidelines, 2010 [1].

Sexual Assault

Sexual assault, defined as any sexual act performed by one person on another without consent, is common. Nearly one in three women in the United States experiences a sexual assault during her lifetime [2]. The prevalence of assault or attempted assault is particularly high in college women; one in four in some surveys [3]. These college-related assaults may take place in the setting of drug or alcohol use, with associated impairment or intoxication of the victim, rather than the classic situation in which force or threats are involved.

C.M. Stroka, DO (✉) • M.M. Clark, MD
Family Medicine Residency Program, Abington Memorial Hospital, 500 Old York Road, Suite 108, Jenkintown, PA 19046, USA
e-mail: cstroka@amh.org

N.S. Skolnik et al. (eds.), *Sexually Transmitted Diseases: A Practical Guide for Primary Care*, Current Clinical Practice, DOI 10.1007/978-1-62703-499-9_13,
© Springer Science+Business Media New York 2013

A minority of sexual assault victims—10–15%—report these assaults to police. This figure is even lower in the roughly half of women who have some acquaintance with their attackers.

How should a clinician respond to a patient who reports a sexual assault? The Centers for Disease Control and Prevention (CDC) and other experts strongly recommend that evaluation be done only by experienced providers, who are specifically trained in this complex aspect of care. If at all possible, patients should be encouraged to seek care at a center which can obtain the necessary forensic evidence, competently assess the medical and psychological issues, and provide comprehensive treatment and follow-up. The Department of Justice supports such training and certification through the Sexual Assault Nurse Evaluation (SANE) program; affiliated centers can be located online [4].

Nevertheless, primary care clinicians may find themselves as the first point of contact for a sexual assault victim, and the patient may choose not to make a police report, or decline evaluation and treatment at a specialty center or emergency department. We present an overview of these issues, so that the clinician can fully appreciate them, and can provide informed guidance to patients as they seek care following a sexual assault.

Forensic Evidence

In order for forensic evidence to be useful in prosecution, the patient should alter as little as possible prior to her examination. Specifically, she should not change clothes, bathe, wipe, change tampons, eat or drink, brush teeth, douche, or use an enema.

Laws vary by state, but as a rule evidence may be legally obtained up to several days following an assault. Evidence collection kits and specific forms should be used, including documentation of chain of custody for any specimens collected [5]. These may be extensive, and include swabs from the mouth, vagina and rectum, blood testing, plucked hair samples, and nail clippings. This evidence, including the clothing worn by the patient at the time of assault, will be saved in police custody.

Victims may expect detailed questioning regarding the assault, including specifics about recent consensual sexual activity.

With the patient's consent, a detailed physical examination is done, with particular attention to areas that involved penetration or trauma, and including appropriate photographic documentation.

Clearly, for someone who has undergone a sexual assault, the process outlined above can be challenging. Most centers experienced in treating sexual assault victims will have advocates and counselors available, to assist the patient as she completes this evaluation, and will make accommodations for the presence of a supportive friend or family.

Testing for STDs

Aside from the forensic considerations detailed above, the CDC recommends the following diagnostic testing in a victim of sexual assault:

- Testing for chlamydia and gonorrhea, preferably with nucleic acid amplification tests (NAATs).
- A wet mount and culture for trichomonas, with the wet mount examined for bacterial vaginosis as well.
- Serum testing for HIV, hepatitis B, and syphilis.

Depending on the time elapsed since the assault took place, initial STD testing may be negative. This is particularly true for hepatitis B and HIV. This leads to recommendations for appropriate repeat testing, and for empiric treatment, as outlined below.

Empiric Treatment of STDs

The CDC recommends routine preventive therapy after a sexual assault. As an alternative, an assault victim could be tested, with treatment being reserved for positive tests or the development of symptoms. However, empiric treatment is favored for two reasons. First, testing is not perfect, and an infection might escape detection. Secondly, compliance with follow-up testing and treatment is poor in victims of sexual assault, so that the initial evaluation may be the best—or only—opportunity for effective treatment. Disease-specific preventive regimens include the following:

Hepatitis B

Postexposure hepatitis B vaccination, in previously unvaccinated women, effectively prevents hepatitis B infection in victims of sexual assault, even if administered after the assault took place. The administration of HBIG is not necessary. Follow-up immunization should be offered (at 1- and 6-month interval) to complete the three-dose series.

Chlamydia, Gonorrhea, and Trichomonas

The CDC recommends empiric antibiotic treatment for all three of these infectious agents, with the following medications:

Ceftriaxone 250 mg IM as a single dose
and
Metronidazole 2 g orally as a single dose
Plus either
Azithromycin 1 g orally as a single dose
Or
Doxycycline 100 mg orally twice a day for 7 days

While the 2010 CDC guidelines also included the option of giving oral cefixime instead of ceftriaxone, this is no longer considered appropriate treatment for gonorrhea, due to increasing patterns of cephalosporin resistance [6].

HIV

While the risk of acquiring HIV from a sexual assault is probably low, the CDC recommends that post-exposure prophylaxis (PEP) with antiviral medication be considered, and discussed with the patient. This recommendation is based on extrapolation from data on HIV transmission in other settings. In consensual sex, the risk for HIV transmission is 0.1–0.2 % for vaginal intercourse, and 0.5–3 % for receptive rectal intercourse. The risk of transmission may be increased in sexual assault victims, particularly if there is mucosal trauma or skin injury. On the other hand, an assailant's HIV status, while usually unknown, would certainly be negative in many cases, so the overall risk of acquiring HIV from an assault would be less than the figures quoted above, which apply to contact with known HIV-positive partners. The specific risk of HIV transmission for a given patient would depend upon information such as the characteristics of the assailant, the sites of penetration, the degree of mucosal injury or bleeding, and the presence of genital lesions.

For PEP to be effective, it should be started within 72 h of the assault. Although the CDC operates a PEP hotline (888-448-4911) to assist with the decision to initiate medication, it is strongly recommended that consultation with an infectious disease specialist be obtained as part of this process.

Emergency Contraception

All victims of sexual assault should be offered emergency contraception. This is particularly true if there is any question that the assault might result in pregnancy (i.e., vaginal penetration and inadequate contraception). The following regimens are currently available for emergency contraception [7].

- Oral contraceptive pills (progestin-only birth control pills or combined estrogen/progesterone contraceptives, commonly referred to as the Yuzpe method)

- Progestin only pill (available as levonorgestrel-containing "Plan B One Step," "Plan B," or "Next Choice")
- Copper IUD (paraGard)
- Ulipristal Acetate (Ella)

The most recent American Congress of Obstetricians and Gynecologists (ACOG) guidelines favor the use of progestin-only regimens over combined OCPs, due to greater efficacy and fewer side effects. The levonorgestrel methods are available to patients and partners 17 years old or more, but younger women need a prescription. Of note, all hormonal emergency contraception is less effective in overweight and obese women than in normal-weight women, and efficacy declines with increasing time since intercourse occurred. The progestin-only methods as well as the combined oral contraceptives are all most effective if started within 72 h of unprotected intercourse.

The copper IUD (paraGuard) is the most expensive yet most effective form of emergency contraception. If inserted within 5 days of unprotected intercourse, it can reduce the risk of pregnancy by 99.9 %. It does, however, require insertion, and may not be covered by insurance.

Ella (ulipristal acetate) is the newest drug approved by the FDA for emergency contraception. It is a selective progesterone receptor modulator and was approved in August 2010. It is a single 30 mg pill taken as soon as possible after unprotected sex or contraception failure for up to 120 h (5 days) after intercourse [8]. Like most emergency contraception methods, it is most effective immediately after unprotected sex but seems to be superior to other levonorgesterol methods in the 72–120 h window. Similar to other hormonal methods, it appears to be less effective in obese women with a BMI >30. Adverse effects are similar to those of levonorgestrel, and include headache, abdominal pain, and nausea.

The cost for emergency contraception varies greatly and depends on the method. Plan B One Step typically costs $35–60; Next Choice is typically somewhat lower. Ella costs around $55, and fees for the ParaGard IUD, including insertion, are typically around $400 [9].

Psychological Evaluation and Support

Women who have been sexually assaulted require emotional support, and should be offered mental health services as soon as possible. Psychological effects vary among victims. Common emotional reactions include fear, anxiety, anger, guilt, shame, and helplessness [10]. The patient should be reassured that these are normal feelings following an assault. Somatic reactions are common and include development of muscle tension, gastrointestinal irritability, dyspareunia, dysuria, and sleep disturbances. Victims often also experience mood swings and irritability and may suffer from PTSD, anxiety, depression, suicidal ideation, and drug abuse/misuse.

Recognizing that the victim is at risk for these problems can allow the primary care physician to direct the patient to the appropriate victim resources.

Unprotected Sexual Contact without Sexual Assault

In cases of sexual contact without protection from pregnancy or STDs (e.g., no condom or other barrier use, and/or inadequate contraception) but where no sexual assault has taken place, the forensic considerations detailed above may not apply. Clinicians should bear in mind, however, that issues of consent may be murky for the patient, particularly if drugs or alcohol were involved, even if these were taken voluntarily. As discussed above, an intoxicated/impaired person is legally unable to give consent, but may assume an assault was her fault. When strong uncertainty exists, referral to a trained rape crisis worker or law enforcement personnel may be appropriate.

Even in situations where no sexual assault has apparently occurred, the above recommendations relating to testing and empiric treatment may still be relevant. Emergency contraception, empiric treatment for gonorrhea, chlamydia, and trichomonas as detailed above, and hepatitis B vaccination may all make sense in this setting. If the partner is known, and willing to provide a medical history and undergo testing, concerns about PEP for HIV infection may be greatly diminished.

Conclusion

Victims of sexual assault present specialized concerns with respect to taking a sensitive and thorough history, obtaining legally binding evidence, making accurate medical diagnoses, and providing appropriate treatment. If at all possible, the patient should be referred to a specialized evaluation and treatment center. Primary care clinicians can help facilitate appropriate care by being informed about what is involved, and by providing the patient with supportive anticipatory guidance.

References

1. Workowski KA, Berman S, Centers for Disease Control and Prevention (CDC). Sexually transmitted diseases treatment guidelines, 2010. MMWR Morb Mortal Wkly Rep. 2010;59:1.
2. Tjaden P, Thoennes N. Extent, nature, and consequences of rape victimization: Findings from the national violence against women survey. Washington, DC: National Institute of Justice; 2006. www.ncjrs.gov/pdffiles1/nij/210346.pdf
3. Fisher BS, Cullen FT, Turner MG. The sexual victimization of college women. Washington, DC: National Institute of Justice; 2000. www.ncjrs.gov/pdffiles1/nij/182369.pdf

4. Ledray LE. SANE development and operation guide. J Emerg Nurs. 1998;24(2):197–8 [PMID: 9775832].
5. A national protocol for sexual assault medical forensic examinations: adults/adolescents, President's DNA Initiative, Office on Violence Against Women, Washington, DC: US Department of Justice: September 2004.
6. Centers for Disease control and Prevention (CDC). Update to CDC's STD treatment guidelines: oral cephalosporins no longer a recommended treatment for gonococcal infections. MMWR Morb Mortal Wkly Rep. 2012;61(31):590–4.
7. American College of Obstetricians and Gynecologists. ACOG Practice Bulletin No. 112: emergency contraception. Obstet Gynecol. 2010;115(5):1100–9 [PubMed PMID: 20410799].
8. Whalen K, Rose R. Ulipristal (Ella) for emergency contraception. Am Fam Physician. 2012;86(4):365, 369. [PubMed PMID: 22963027].
9. Armstrong C. ACOG recommendations on emergency contraception. Am Fam Physician. 2010;82(10):1278 [PubMed PMID: 21121541].
10. Brown AL, Testa M, Messman-Moore TL. Psychological consequences of sexual victimization resulting from force, incapacitation, or verbal coercion. Violence Against Women. 2009;15:898–919.

Index